MILADY'S AESTHETICIAN SERIES

Advanced Face and
Body Treatments for the Spa

MILADY'S AESTHETICIAN SERIES

Advanced Face and Body Treatments for the Spa

PAMELA HILL, R.N.

LAURA TODD

THOMSON

DELMAR LEARNING

Australia Canada Mexico Singapore Spain United Kingdom United States

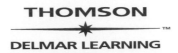

THOMSON

DELMAR LEARNING

Milady's Aesthetician Series: Advanced Face and Body Treatments for the Spa
Pamela Hill and Laura Todd

President, Milady:
Dawn Gerrain

Managing Editor:
Robert L. Serenka

Acquisitions Editor:
Martine Edwards

Product Manager:
Jessica Burns

Editorial Assistant:
Falon Ferraro

Director of Content and Media Production:
Wendy A. Troeger

Content Project Manager:
Nina Tucciarelli

Composition:
Pre-PressPMG

Director of Marketing:
Wendy Mapstone

Director Beauty Industry Relations:
Sandra Bruce

Marketing Coordinator:
Nicole Riggi

Text Design:
Essence of Seven

Library of Congress Cataloging-in-Publication Data
Hill, Pamela, RN.
    Advanced face and body treatments for the spa / Pamela Hill, Laura Todd.
        p. ; cm. -- (Milady's aesthetician series)
    Includes bibliographical references and index.
    ISBN-13: 978-1-4018-8175–7
    1. Skin--Care and hygiene. 2. Beauty, Personal. 3. Beauty shops. I. Todd, Laura (Laura A.), 1967- . II. Title.
    RL87.H55 2008
    646.7'26--dc22
                                    2007024151

NOTICE TO THE READER

Publisher does not warrant or guarantee any of the products described herein or perform any independent analysis in connection with any of the product information contained herein. Publisher does not assume, and expressly disclaims, any obligation to obtain and include information other than that provided to it by the manufacturer.

The reader is expressly warned to consider and adopt all safety precautions that might be indicated by the activities herein and to avoid all potential hazards. By following the instructions contained herein, the reader willingly assumes all risks in connection with such instructions.

The Publisher makes no representation or warranties of any kind, including but not limited to, the warranties of fitness for particular purpose or merchantability, nor are any such representations implied with respect to the material set forth herein, and the publisher takes no responsibility with respect to such material. The publisher shall not be liable for any special, consequential, or exemplary damages resulting, in whole or part, from the readers' use of, or reliance upon, this material.

Contents

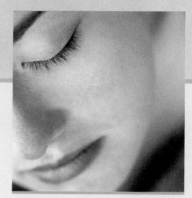

■ **CHAPTER 5**

Preface

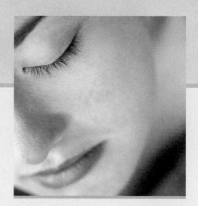

The spa and the medical spa were once specific concepts that did not intermingle. But, as the industry has evolved, both of these client care models have blossomed and are now frequently intermingled. Many times neither the client nor the aesthetician has any idea that this is happening. Today, it is not uncommon to find medical treatments such as Botox in the day spa and treatments such as body wraps in the medical spa. It has become a fusion of ideas and treatments.

This book builds on these concepts, focusing on advanced face and body treatments that can be provided for clients. Rather than having a medical bent, these treatments focus on the relaxation and pampering necessary in our busy world. While not proper medical care, these treatments certainly impact the well-being of the individuals who are treated.

The chapters are built one on top of the next, focusing on the anatomy and physiology of the skin first and then moving to the muscular and cardiovascular systems. A relaxing treatment can obviously affect these systems and the aesthetician should have a good understanding of what the results could and should be when providing certain treatments.

Many treatments included in this text will be familiar, such as facials. But other treatments such as lymphatic drainage are new to a textbook such as this and contain cutting-edge information. Finally, as always, there is information about marketing your spa and a chapter on how to run your spa is also included. It is a complete guide for providing the most imaginative and progressive treatments. As our industry continues to fight for its identity and the concepts continue to change, a textbook such as this one is essential for learning and continuing to compete in today's spa world.

About the Authors

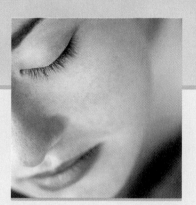

Pamela Hill received her nursing diploma from Presbyterian Hospital and Colorado Women's College, Denver, Colorado, and has practiced as a registered nurse for more than 20 years. Her background includes 15 years of operational and leadership experience in the medical spa, medical skin care, and educational sector. Ms. Hill has been instrumental in the growth and development of Facial Aesthetics, Inc. ("FAI"), a successful Colorado-based medical spa. An astute results-oriented leader with a proven track record of building and growing companies in the medical appearance sector, she has been actively involved in the evolution of the medical spa model as well as the research and development of the Pamela Hill Skin Care product line. Ms. Hill has been active with patient care, the development of policy and procedure, and clinician education. Passionate about the education of aestheticians in the medical spa setting, Ms. Hill began a relationship with Milady, an imprint of Thomson Delmar Learning, in 2003. This relationship launched Ms. Hill's authoring of the Aesthetician Series, a 12-book series dedicated to the education of medical aestheticians and the must-have information for on-the-job success. Currently six of the books are in print.

Laura Todd has been in the esthetics industry for more than 20 years, earning national attention and commendation. She holds a Bachelor's degree in Science with a minor in Biology and is a Master's degree candidate. Currently, Laura is the president of the Institute of Advanced Medical Esthetics and the University of Professional Sciences in Richmond, Virginia. She is also a practicing medical esthetician at her medispa, Spa Rx.

Laura has been an active participant in advocating for and implementing current legislation to establish licensure for estheticians in the state of Virginia. Laura holds Virginia's first full-term Esthetician Seat, appointed by the governor, and serves on the board that regulates esthetics in Virginia. She was an integral part of developing state regulations for esthetics education, which has influenced policy in other states as well as national legislation. Laura has also served as a subject matter expert, assisting in the development of Virginia's master esthetician examination and the national master esthetician examination for NIC.

Acknowledgments

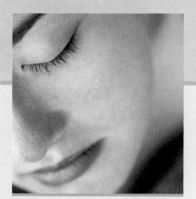

Pamela Hill

As mothers we recognize the beauty of life. My daughter Alysa has shown me that being pampered is not such a bad thing. In fact, it is necessary for today's way of life. The best part of being spa pampered is having treatments together. So, here is to many more years of being spa pampered together, Alysa.

I would also like to thank Laura Todd, my co-author for all the work and research that she put into this textbook. The book you hold in your hands would not be the work it is without Laura's hard work. Thank you, Laura, for the late nights, the research, and the help you contributed to make this such a great book.

Laura Todd

I would like to thank my family for the support they offered me during this project; without their support, I would not be where I am today. I would also like to thank Christine Gordon for being a great mentor and friend.

Most of all, I would like to thank Pamela Hill for the opportunity to work on this project and for all of her encouragement and guidance. Pamela, if it were not for your knowledge, influence and valuable textbooks, this industry would not be where it is today. As a school owner myself, I cannot stress how valuable this book is and how it will help educators impart the necessary knowledge to mold future estheticians.

Milady and the authors would like to thank the following for contributing to this series:

Christine Gordon, President of International Education Group, Graham Webb Academy, for hosting our photo shoot at her school in Arlington, VA

Larry Hamill Photography, Columbus, OH

Christine A. Clinton, International Spa & Salon Services

Elena L. Reichel, PR and Partners

Manufacturers and suppliers who have graciously provided products for use during the photo shoot:

Circadia Skincare from Dr. Peter T. Pugliese

ilike organic skin care from szép élet, LLC

Models who participated in the photo shoot:

Anastasia Arnold
Julianne Baddock
Robin Carlson
Randi Engel
Swaroopa Giangapathy
Isabella Gomez
Michaela Hulgaard
Courtney Hungerford
Jenna McDonald
Tram Nguyen
Lisa Nyden
Janice Ricketts
Barry Smithers
Sarah Tope
Jenny Vo
Kim Williams
Tania Williams

Photo credits

All location photographs provided by Larry Hamill Photography, Columbus, Ohio

Chapter 1: Figure 1–4: Photograph courtesy of Facial Aesthetics

Chapter 2: Figure 2–2: Fitzpatrick et al., Color Atlas and Synopsis of Clinical Dermatology 3E, 1997. Reprinted with the permission of The McGraw-Hill Companies

Chapter 7: Figure 7–8: Photo courtesy of Randall Perry Photography

Chapter 8: Figure 8–8: Courtesy of Syneron

Reviewers

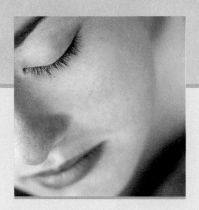

The authors and publisher would like to thank the following individuals who have reviewed this text and offered invaluable feedback. This very important task, although time consuming for each reviewer, is a critical component to the success of a book. We are grateful for your time and honest comments.

Sheryl Baba,
Owner, Solstice Day Spa, Cape Cod, MA

Felicia Brown, LMBT,
Spalutions!, Beyond Bodywork Solutions, Greensboro, NC

Kathy Hernandez, L.Ac. Dipl. Ac.,
San Bernardino, CA

Tracy Johnson, RN, LE,
Wingate Salon & Spa, Stratham, NH

Cheryl McDonald, BSVE,
Credential (Life) Cosmetology and Barbering,
Solano Community College, Fairfield, CA

Elizabeth Myron,
General Manager, Hive Beauty USA

Ada Polla Tray, MBA,
President, Alchimie Forever LLC

Introduction to Body Wraps

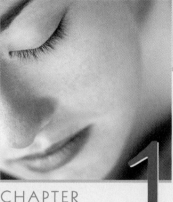

CHAPTER

1

KEY TERMS

balneology

balneotherapy

bloodborne pathogens

Bloodborne Pathogens
  Act

career plan

Centers for Disease
  Control and Prevention
  (CDC)

disinfection

hepatitis

herpes simplex

HIV/AIDS

hydrotherapy

Langelier Index

Mission Statement

OSHA

pH

sanitas per aquas

sterilization

technique sensitive

training

training protocol

vichy shower

water testing

waterborne infections

LEARNING OBJECTIVES

After completing this chapter, you should be able to:

1. Discuss the global evolution of spa treatments.

2. Discuss the popularity of spas in the United States.

3. Explore the history and origins of spa treatments and water therapies.

4. Establish the importance of training and how to evaluate clinical skills.

5. Discuss the importance of OSHA, safety, and cleanliness in the spa.

1

INTRODUCTION

The goal of spa treatments is to affect the whole body, inducing a physical and mental sense of well-being. (See Table 1–1.) Typically a spa atmosphere is meant to relax the client and is very different from clinical or medical settings that get so much attention today. There are certain benefits of a spa treatment, among them a sense of pleasure and well-being. However, it should not be misunderstood that spa treatments, as we know them in the United States, are long term medicinal treatment processes for any serious medical condition. Those conditions should be treated by the physician and, if appropriate and agreed upon with the physician, augmented with spa treatments. The type of spa (resort, day spa, cruise ship) and the treatments offered will vary from facility to facility and will depend on the space that is available, the equipment, and the capabilities of the aestheticians. Spa services generally require more space as well as showers and wet rooms. In fact, when using the word "spa" to identify a service or establishment, it implies that some type of water or mud therapy is offered. (See Table 1–2.)

There are several important considerations that should be addressed when the spa is moving into advanced treatments, beyond just facials and waxing, for example. First, a menu should be considered. Development of a menu is a business decision that requires thought, financial planning, and market investigation. As this process progresses, it will become clear what equipment is needed. Adding advanced treatments will require specialized equipment that can be expensive and dedicated to a single service; an example of this might be a **vichy shower**. Finally, it is important to understand that the qualifications and capabilities of an aesthetician can be critical to the overall success of a spa offering advanced treatments. More about this subject will be covered in our final chapter of this text.

vichy shower
an overhead shower with adjustable water pressure used in body treatments

Table 1–1 Spa Treatments	
What the Treatments Can Do	**What the Treatment Cannot Do**
Give a sense of pleasure and relaxation	Provide lasting improvements
Provide a relaxing atmosphere	
Temporarily improve the appearance of the skin	Treat serious medical conditions
Temporarily revitalize the spirit	Treat psychiatric conditions

Table 1–2   Different Types of Spa Treatments
Body Scrubs
Hydrotherapy Tub Treatments
Sauna and Steam Treatments
Body Wraps
Facials
Waxing or Laser Hair Removal
Makeup Applications
Brow and Lash Tinting, Lash Perming
Manicures and Pedicures
Massages
Aromatherapy Treatments
Reflexology Treatments
Lymphatic Drainage

The Global Evolution of Spas and Spa Treatments

Understanding the history of the spa and spa treatments is especially important. It helps the aesthetician to know the purpose of the treatment and how the treatment evolved. Let us take a look at the history and evolution of the spa industry.

The origin of the word "spa" has several possibilities. One theory is that the word "spa" may be derived from the Walloon word "espa," which means fountain and originates from the name of the Belgian town Spa. Other possibilities are that "spa" is an acronym of the Latin phrase "**sanitas per aquas**" (health through water) or that it originates from the Latin word "spagere" (to scatter, sprinkle, moisten). All origins communicate the process, the use of water, and the implication for healing. The water treatments provided in the spa are defined as **balneotherapy**, spa therapy, and hydrotherapy and can be used interchangeably.

While many spa treatments seem new and never before tried, the reality is that most of the spa treatments we provide today are derivations of ancient treatments. It is thought that spa treatments began with

sanitas per aquas
(health through water) originates from the Latin word "spagere" (to scatter, sprinkle, moisten)

balneotherapy
along with spa therapy and hydrotherapy, balneotherapy involves the use of baths from the sea water, freshwater, or thermal springs, and may include drinking the water

bathhouses in ancient Greece and Roman Empire times. Originally the Roman bathing culture had a medicinal focus before evolving toward the use of baths for relaxation. There were three types of bathhouses in Rome: balnea (home), balnea private (private baths), and balnea public (public baths). Known for their vast aqueducts, the Romans created enormous bathhouses on their newly conquered lands where baths were combined with other healthy endeavors such as exercise and massage. When the Roman Empire fell, only a few of the original bathhouses escaped destruction. During this time, public bathing was prohibited by the Christian culture; in fact, some people would avoid bathing for years. Most bathhouses were turned into churches since prayer was considered more important than relaxation.

In the thirteenth century, the Moors had great influence in Southern Europe. This contributed to a resurgence in bathing and in public bath popularity. Again, bathing was primarily for the purpose of relaxation. But medicinal processes such as bloodletting were also performed at the baths.

The sixteenth century and the Renaissance period saw a decline in public baths again. The decline was due to many factors, including the lack of firewood to heat the bathhouse and water, as well as the hypothesis that the bathhouse was the cause for diseases such as syphilis and leprosy. Nevertheless, the wealthy continued to visit bathhouses, though they preferred baths of natural sources such as hot springs or mineral water.

During this time, natural mineral springs gained popularity. A scientific attempt was made to analyze the water's mineral content to try to establish if there was any therapeutic value in **balneology**. At this time, the philosophy of drinking the water as well as bathing in the water became commonplace. The first bath was used for drinking, while the second bath was used for bathing. Through these efforts the benefits of mud therapy were acknowledged and elite Italians began to enjoy these luxuries.

During the seventeenth century, the French joined the movement. They used hot and cold springs. Cold springs were used only for drinking therapies while the hot springs were used for drinking cures as well as bathing. These therapies were taken quite seriously, and at this time the physician became an integral part of the spa experience in France.

In the 1800s a more scientific approach was taken as attempts to replicate natural mineral springs' benefits for medicinal purposes were made. A Bavarian monk, Father Sebastian Kneipp, believed that disease could be cured by using water to eliminate waste from the body. He developed over 100 different hydrotherapy treatments using water in solid, liquid,

balneology
the study of spa therapy, hydrotherapy involving the use of baths from the sea water, freshwater, or thermal springs

and vapor forms to treat individuals. His treatments included washings, wraps, packs, compresses, steam, and baths.

When Europeans began to immigrate to America, they brought the spa concept with them, which resulted in an increase in the number of spas seen in the United States. The trend was to develop hotels and guest houses around mineral springs. This movement led to what was known as spa resorts. These resorts, which also included theaters and casinos, were very popular with both the elite and middle classes.

When the Depression hit in the 1930s, the development of spas halted in the United States. Many European spas that had catered to Americans were closed. But after World War II and with the economy on the rise spas became popular again. This time treatments, such as health and exercise regiments, mud therapy, balneology, and **hydrotherapy**, were added. But eventually the focus of a preventive practice lost ground with the advances of modern medicine. Spas were once again on the decline.

hydrotherapy
the use of water in treatments

Today, there is a spa revival worldwide that recognizes the benefits of preventative therapies.[1] Spas have become an important component of American life, becoming one of the fastest growing industries in the United States. According to ISPA's latest statistics, spas generated $11.2 billion in a single year. The American public is flocking to spas for rejuvenation, relaxation, therapeutic treatments, and much more.

The Popularity of Spas in the United States

Today's spas have evolved to offer a wide variety of services in multiple settings. Day spas, cruise ship spas, destination spas, resort spas, and medical spas provide clients respite, relaxation, and therapeutic treatments.

Between 1977 and 2002, the salon/spa industry sales grew a strong 41 percent—well above the 26 percent increase in the United States' gross domestic product during the same five-year period. The salon/spa industry is projected to add nearly 86,000 jobs by 2012, which is a 15 percent increase.[2]

European Thermal Spas

European spas remain focused on water therapy more so than their American counterparts. Some Europeans even use the term "thermal waters" when describing a spa. There is an accepted belief in Europe that these "thermal waters" have a noticeable effect on motor skills, skin, mental health, and other conditions. Thermal waters are thought to be useful as a homeopathic alternative to drugs or surgery.

training
an educational course designed to
complete a clearly defined objective

technique sensitive
a procedure that is performed
differently from aesthetician to
aesthetician based on his or her
experience and knowledge

▪ TRAINING

Training is understood to be a requisite component of all spa related procedures. Aestheticians receive a solid educational foundation when they attend school that is general in nature, allowing them to adapt to any product line or basic treatment protocol. Typically spas have treatment protocols that are specific or proprietary in nature, known as signature treatments. Employers are looking for aestheticians who are willing to comply with their company's vision and protocols to ensure customer satisfaction. This element of treatment repetition and adherence to protocol is important to the image of the spa and for client retention. (See Figure 1–1.)

Imagine if every time you visited your favorite restaurant the dish you looked forward to was prepared a different way. Most successful businesses are successful because of consistent quality. Reliability is important. This is where advanced training comes into the picture.

Each spa has a menu of services that it offers, and training ensures that each practitioner is delivering the same quality and standard for each procedure. Because the advanced spa treatments could be touch and **technique sensitive**, the aesthetician must be educated to under-

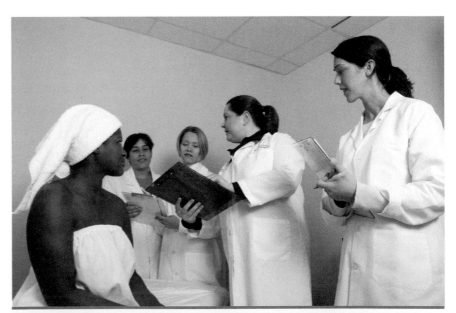

Figure 1–1 Training is understood to be a requisite component of all spa related procedures

stand the purpose for the order of the treatment steps. Furthermore, knowledge of the anatomy and physiology of the skin, muscles, and cardiovascular system, as well as proper management for aftercare, are important factors for the overall success of the treatment. (See Figure 1–2.)

The training process for advanced spa treatments should not be left to the product vendor. Rather the vendor is a good resource of information about how his or her product will behave on the skin and the potential outcome. The treatment itself should become a signature of the spa, designed and developed by the spa. That said, the depth of knowledge

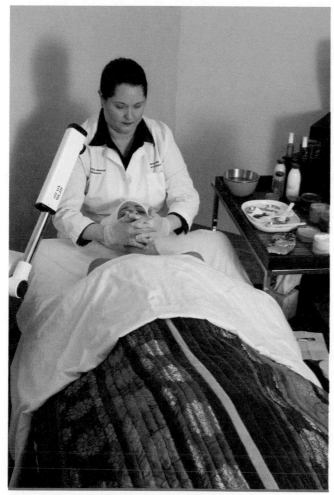

Figure 1–2 Knowledge of the anatomy and physiology of the skin, muscles, and cardiovascular system is important when doing a facial

necessary to be successful in advanced spa treatments cannot be satisfactorily achieved with a vendor educator.

Training Protocols

training protocol
a standard that is developed to ensure
that a treatment is performed properly

A **training protocol** is a set standard that is developed to ensure that a treatment is performed within the parameters set forth by the facility and that the treatment can be duplicated by all practitioners, achieving the same results for each client. A training protocol outlines who can be trained, how long the training will take place, how many models need to be treated prior to working with actual clients, and who will conduct the training. These protocols ensure that quality services are delivered and safety is practiced. Having these protocols in place can protect the facility from liability. Protocols should be reviewed and updated on a yearly basis, or sooner, if needed.

Typically a senior staff member or a spa educator provides the training for new employees.

To ensure that the aesthetician is properly trained for advanced spa procedures, a classroom session should precede any treatment room lesson. The content of this classroom session should include anatomy and physiology of the skin, muscles, and cardiovascular system. Each of these body systems is affected during an advanced spa treatment. Some treatments will require more information about a particular body system and some less. The level of information taught will depend on the treatment procedure lesson. Nevertheless, review of these three body systems should not be skipped. Once this information has been reviewed, the essence of the treatment should be discussed, including the proper candidate for the treatment, those who are contraindicated for the treatment, the steps of the treatment, and the recommended take-home products. Once this classroom training has been completed, the training moves to the treatment room. The first treatment should be provided by the instructor to an employee other than the student. This way, the student can observe the treatment and learn the steps. Next, it is the student's turn to provide a treatment. Typically, models are abundant and providing training treatments is not a problem. (See Figure 1–3.)

During spa training, an aesthetician should be required to complete a specified number of treatments according to the company's specific protocol. This should be accomplished before being allowed to work on clients. There should also be training in documentation and recommended products to take after the treatment is complete. At the end of training the aesthetician should be tested to ensure that he or she can perform the duties without direct supervision.

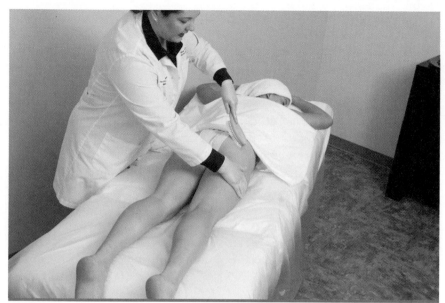

Figure 1–3 Body treatments will require more knowledge about the muscles and cardiovascular system of the body

■ THE OCCUPATIONAL SAFETY AND HEALTH ADMINISTRATION

The Occupational Safety and Health Act (29 U.S.C. 651 ET SEQ) was created by the Department of Labor in an effort to reduce on-the-job hazards. This act requires that all employers provide safe working conditions and that training programs be developed and implemented to increase competency and safety for personnel. The Occupational Safety and Health Administration (**OSHA**) is authorized to conduct workplace inspections without advance notification, to determine if there are any noncompliance issues and to impose penalties on the employer when appropriate. OSHA also provides guidelines on record keeping, sterilization, disinfection, housekeeping, and labeling requirements. Nationally governed, OSHA's laws supersede state laws.

OSHA has many rules and regulations, far too many for us to cover in this small section. However, it is necessary for us to discuss the rules of OSHA that generally apply to the spa and spa treatments, such as **bloodborne pathogens** and the use of Universal Precautions. The protocol we will be concerning ourselves with should be outlined specifically in your spa's safety manual.

OSHA
the Occupational Safety and Health Administration

bloodborne pathogens
any pathogens that can be transmitted through blood or bodily fluids

The Occupational Safety and Health Administration (OSHA) was originally known as the Safety Bill of Rights. It was developed by the federal government to protect workers, initially those in hazardous work environments.

The **Bloodborne Pathogens Act** is part of the OSHA rules and laws. It was legally enforceable as of July 5, 1992, and was initiated to reduce the transmission of **hepatitis** B and other bloodborne pathogens. One component of this regulation is the requirement that employers make available the hepatitis B vaccine if employees are at risk of potential exposure to the virus. If the employees forego the vaccination, they must sign a declination statement that must be maintained in their records.

The **Centers for Disease Control and Prevention (CDC)** has a recommended policy regarding blood and bodily fluids called Universal Precautions. The primary goal of this policy is to educate workers on how to reduce the risk of exposure to bloodborne pathogens by using personal protective equipment such as gloves, protective clothing, and face shields.

Infectious diseases are spread via direct contact through skin or mucous membranes. Aestheticians in the spa setting can come in contact with mucous membranes, possibly skin lesions, blood, and body fluid.

The subject of using gloves is controversial and has simmered among aestheticians for many years. Many aestheticians think that it is acceptable to wear gloves only during extractions or during facial treatments. Nothing could be further from the truth. When anyone has direct physical contact with another person during a clinical treatment, gloves should be used. Some aestheticians have justified the absence of gloves since massage therapists, hair dressers, and nail techs do not wear gloves. Justifying that opinion based on what others do not do is untenable.

Hepatitis B, C, and HIV may require intimate contact with bodily fluids, but we should not be focused only on these diseases. Some individuals carry bad bacteria on the surface of their skin. Examples of these are MRSA, Salmonella, or *E. Coli.* We normally wash our hands before treating a client. But if you treat a client without gloves, consider this: some individuals are more fastidious than others. What about the persons who do not wash their hands after using the toilet and then touch their face or nose? What about their hands? Are their face and hands contaminated with Salmonella or *E. Coli?* Probably. After treating this client, do you wash your hands before touching your face or someone else for that matter? Do you ensure that you wash your hands thoroughly, cleaning under the fingernails and cuticles with a brush or pick using a medical antibacterial soap? If we are to be true professionals, we need to consider gloves a required part of our business attire.

Wearing gloves (which provide a protective barrier for individuals who have lesions or dermatitis) during all treatments, from start to finish, and following the strictest sterilization procedures, including Universal Precautions, to prevent the spread of infectious agents are important for the safety of all involved.[3]

Disinfection

Spa treatments involve heat and moisture, providing an ideal environment for the breeding of harmful microorganisms. It is important that all furnishings are regularly cleaned and disinfected as recommended by the manufacturers.

It is also important to always follow strict standards and to treat every client as if he or she could be carrying an infection. Always wear gloves during all treatments. All implements that are used should be properly disinfected, sterilized, or disposed. Any object that has been touched requires disinfection.

It is important to remember the difference between sterilization and disinfection. **Sterilization** is the destruction of all microbial life by heat, chemical stimulant, or gas. **Disinfection** eliminates pathogenic microorganisms on inanimate objects, except for bacterial spores.[4]

sterilization
the destruction of all microbial life by heat, chemical, or gas

disinfection
eliminates pathogenic microorganisms on inanimate objects (except for bacterial spores)

After Each Client's Visit

1. Remove any dirty spatulas, used brushes, tools, implements, or other materials and disinfect.
2. Wear gloves at all times.
3. Wash with antibacterial soap and dry with a clean towel.
4. Soak in EPA, hospital-grade disinfectant for 10 to 20 minutes (according to manufacturer's instructions). Remember to change the disinfecting solution as necessary. The general rule for this is every two hours or when it gets cloudy.
5. Rinse, towel dry, and store in closed nonairtight container.
6. Bowls, electrodes, machines, and counters should be sprayed with an EPA, hospital-grade disinfectant and allowed to set for 10 minutes (or according to manufacturer's instructions). Wipe, repeat, rinse, and towel dry.
7. Other items: Clean any items touched while working on a client with the above procedures. If any bottles are touched while working on a client, they must also be disinfected.[5]

Daily Shutdown Procedures

These following procedures ensure that a spa's treatment rooms are ready in the morning. They also cut down on the number of micro-organisms that can breed in the rooms overnight. Additionally, these procedures keep rooms spotless, which assure clients that they are being treated in a sanitary environment.

1. Wear gloves during the shutdown process.
2. Remove laundry from hamper, wash with chlorine bleach, and dry immediately. Spray hamper with disinfectant spray or wipe down with disinfectant.
3. Wipe down the following with a wet sanitizer/disinfectant: counters, treatment tables, machinery, and furniture.
4. Replenish the following supplies: linens, spatulas, and other disposable items. Replenish empty jars, but always use their entire contents before doing so. Never add cream to a partially used jar. Use gloves when transferring materials. All supplies should be stored in closed containers to prevent contamination prior to use.
5. Clean off dirt, dust, and smudges on walls, baseboards, and air vents and in corners, as well.
6. Vacuum and mop with a disinfectant. Spray room with a disinfecting aerosol spray.[6]

Waterborne Infections

waterborne infections can be acquired in the spa if precautions to prevent the spread of pathogens are not taken

Waterborne infections can be acquired in a spa if precautions to prevent the spread of pathogens are not taken. Methods of entry include superficial trauma before or during a treatment, absorption through undisturbed skin, ingestion, or inhalation. It is advisable not to receive treatments when you have skin lesions. Recently California health officials advised patrons not to shave prior to pedicure services. Methods of precaution include frequent changing and testing of water reservoirs, hand washing, and sterilization of equipment and tools.

In 2005, there was an outbreak of infections that caused lesions on the legs of clients who received pedicure services in California. The lesions were linked to bacteria from contaminated whirlpool footbaths. Local authorities advised clients to avoid shaving their legs before appointments due to nicks and cuts, which are gateways for bacteria. It was also advised that clients with broken skin or lesions on their lower legs refrain from getting pedicures.[7]

Pathogens of concern include fungal infections, herpes simplex virus, and mycobacteria, gram-positive bacteria. The presence of *Escherichia coli* and other fecal coliforms have also been detected in hydrotherapy or hot tubs. *P. aeruginosa,* also known as hot tub folliculitis, *E. rhusiopathiae* (Rosenbach's disease), and seabather's eruption, are conditions that can be acquired through unsanitary conditions and may or may not require antimicrobial therapy.

There are other, more dangerous pathogens that can result in infections requiring treatment with oral or intravenous antibiotics. Gram-negative bacilli, the most common cause of infection, can lead to bacteremia, sepsis, and death as a result of an acute rapidly progressing cellulitis. Treatments for these include multiple intravenous antibiotics for three to four weeks, or longer, and surgical debridement. Mycobacteria, which includes *M. fortuitum, M. marinum,* and *M. ulcerans,* and the fungus *L. loboi* can lead to chronic skin infections and may require a course of three to twelve months of antibiotic treatment and surgical intervention.[8]

Water Testing

Spa attendants, or the individuals who are responsible for maintaining sanitary conditions, should be properly trained and follow the protocol set forth by the spa. When purchasing your equipment, you will find that many manufacturers offer some guidance with the safety protocols that need to be followed, and your local health departments will also be able to provide you with information regarding standards that need to be followed in your state. Additionally, each facility should have written protocols to follow. These written instructions (e.g., the need for a thorough shower prior to a pool or hydrotherapy tub entry) should be displayed in the appropriate treatment areas.

It should be mandatory that a spa's staff make regular safety checks to ensure that the facilities are clean and safe. The facility should have a list of items to check. This checklist should be easy to follow and contain clear instructions on how to rectify any deficiencies noted.

When conducting **water testing**, it is common to test the temperature, hardness (calcium content), **pH** (acidity/alkalinity), and amount of free chlorine that is available to neutralize the water's contaminants, as well as any other chemicals that may be added. The pH is a measure of how acidic, or basic, the water is. The pH scale is a logarithmic one from 0 to 14, with 7 being neutral. Levels below 7 are defined as being acidic. Levels above 7 are defined as being alkaline.

The level of alkalinity in the water is a measurement of all the carbonates, bicarbonates, hydroxides, and other alkaline substances. These substances act as buffers, affecting any potential pH changes. High levels of

water testing
evaluates the temperature, hardness (calcium content), pH (acidity/alkalinity), and amount of free chlorine that is available to neutralize contaminants in the water, as well as any other chemicals that may be added

pH
a measure of the potential of hydrogen that is used to describe the level of acidity or alkalinity

Langelier Index
(or the saturation index) is a chemical equation that is used to diagnose the water balance and includes testing the water for pH, temperature, calcium hardness, and total alkalinity

calcium carbonate also lead to scale buildup. Measuring the concentration of carbonate ions tests the water's softness or hardness.

The saturation index is also known as the **Langelier Index**, which is a chemical equation that is used to diagnose the water balance and includes testing the water for pH, temperature, calcium hardness, and total alkalinity. Typically accepted levels for a spa pool include:

- pH: 7.2–7.8
- Chlorine: 1.0–2.0 ppm
- Total alkalinity: 80–120 ppm
- Calcium hardness: 180–220 ppm (some say 200–400)
- Cyanuric acid: 25–50 ppm
- Total dissolved solids: 500–5000 ppm

Water testing should be conducted according to schedule to ensure patron safety. In commercial facilities it is usually required every hour and must be fully documented. It is common practice for the health department to require that authorized persons carry out all tests and that a record of the tests be maintained for inspection.

OSHA also provides guidelines on record keeping, sterilization, disinfection, housekeeping, and labeling requirements. (See Table 1–3.)

The Bloodborne Pathogens Act, legally enforceable as of July 5, 1992, was initiated to reduce the transmission of hepatitis B and other bloodborne pathogens.

OSHA requires that employers make available the hepatitis B vaccine if employees are at risk of potential exposure to the virus.

OHSA is important because it protects employees' interests and ensures that they have a safe work environment, access to training, and personal protective equipment.

Evaluating Clinician Skills

While written testing is a great tool to evaluate the student through the treatment-related educational process, it is not always an accurate indicator of the clinician's true clinical abilities. In other words, a clinician may be adept at performing the chemical peel treatments, but he or she will

Table 1–3   Why OSHA Is Important to You
The Occupational Safety and Health Act (29 U.S.C. 651 ET SEQ) was created by the Department of Labor as an effort to reduce on-the-job hazards.
This act requires that all employers provide safe working conditions and that training programs be developed and implemented to increase competency and safety of personnel.

Facial Aesthestics Procedure Training and Certification

Date of Origination: June 1996

Creator: Pamela Hill, R.N.

Date of Review: June 1997

Revisions by: S. Smith, M.E.

Date of Revisions: June '98, June '99, June '00, June '01, June '02, June '03

Policy #: 04-001

Attachments: Policy and Procedure Document for Hydrotherapy, Certificates of Completion, Written Test, Clinical Test

Title of Policy: Training and Certification for Hydrotherapy

Policy: All clinical staff will be licensed and insured in the state of employment. Certification through the company training program is required prior to patient care.

Purpose: To ensure that all clinical staff employed by the company are properly trained and certified in the techniques, policies, and procedures through the company training programs

Scope: All clinical personnel

Definition: Clinical Aesthetic Personnel

Procedure Indications: All clinicians seeking certification will be recommended to the training program by their supervisors.

Procedure Contraindications: Not applicable

Required Paperwork: "Recommendation for Training # PER- 43" signed by the clinician supervisor

Testing if Necessary: Score of 80 percent or greater on the written examination is required before proceeding to clinical training. A score of 90 percent or greater on the clinical examination is required to treat patients.

Required Reading: Articles and technical information, provided by the instructor

Classroom Training: The training will consist of two classroom days. The curriculum for these days includes a review of anatomy and physiology of the skin, musculature system, and cardiovascular system. Also included are the principles and techniques of hydrotherapy and recommended home products for use after this procedure. A written test will be administered at the conclusion of the two-day classroom course. A score of at least 80 percent is required to move to the clinical training.

Clinical Training: The clinician will be responsible for finding five models on whom to practice the treatment.

Clinician Requirements: Licensed professional

Clinician Required Training: prerequisite of primary licensure

also need to be reviewed on the nonclinical aspects of performing in the clinic. A simple checklist for the clinician and the clinical instructor might be useful. This *skill list* should include tasks such as draping the client, patient communication skills, home program evaluation, and the ability to orient to the physical space. These skill sets and those identified in Table 1–4 will help the clinician to expand his or her knowledge.

Table 1–4	Additional Clinician Skills	
Clinical Skills	**Score 1–10**	**Recommended Improvements**
Communications Skill		
Clarity		
Education		
Sales		
Safety Skills		
Wears protective gear		
Products		
Understands product lines		
Professionalism		
Appropriate to patient		
Appropriate to peers		

> Ongoing education is the most important thing you will do for your career. It is your annuity for increasing wages, improving treatment results, and realizing self-improvement.

> Ongoing training should be part of a yearly "self-improvement" plan. After you graduate from school, plan to take at least one course a year about a new subject that will add depth and power to your resume.

career plan
a plan used to describe one's professional career goals and how to achieve those goals

Continuing Education

Continuing education is a professional obligation and privilege. While most states do not require yearly documented education for the aesthetician, taking classes each year is an important objective for your career. Keeping up on the newest technology, whether or not you provide the treatment, makes you an educated and knowledgeable aesthetician. Those who are knowledgeable are considered to be authorities by clients and colleagues alike.

■ EMPLOYMENT OPTIONS

Creating a **career plan** for success is the first step to realizing your dream. Many professionals in the area of "self-improvement" recommend identifying the goal and working backward to achieve that goal. (See Table 1–5.)

Using this technique, identify where you want to be in five years and what you want to be doing. Then create a list of objectives to achieve the goal. For example, if you want to get a job as an aesthetician in a resort spa, identify the objectives that will allow you to meet the goal. Find out where to gain the training, expertise, and experience that will allow you to be a valued employee in that spa setting. Identify internships or learning situations that will help you to perfect your skills. Take communication

Table 1–5	Career Opportunities in the Spa Industry
Spas	• Salon Spas • Fitness Club Spas • Country Club Spas • Holistic Spas • Day Spas
Resorts	• Destination Spas • Resort/ Hotel Spas • Cruise Ship Spas • Connoisseur Spas

courses that will help you to learn how to communicate with clients and colleagues in a positive manner. Take sales courses that will help you to make a contribution to your employer and to yourself. Learn the basics of building a business. Create a professional resume. Practice interviewing skills that will help you to get the job.

Marketing yourself to a business will become an important skill for acquiring the right job. Whether you want to land a job in a destination spa, day spa, or a cruise ship spa, the tactics you use to get there will be the same. (See Figures 1–4 and 1–5.) Remember, just as you are looking for

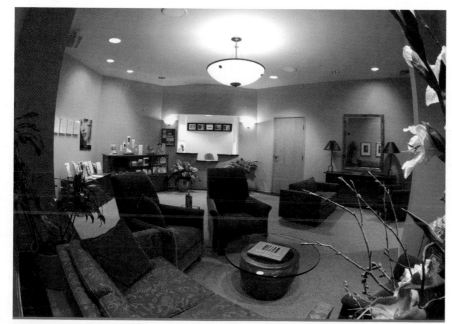

Figure 1–4 A career opportunity might include a medical spa

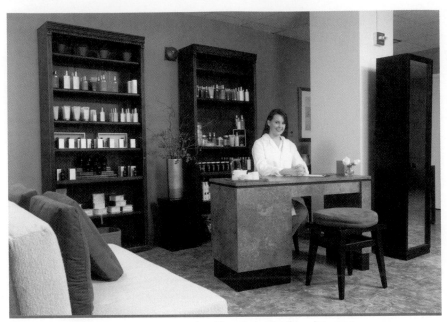

Figure 1–5 Many career opportunities exist in the day spa

the perfect job, the employer is looking for the perfect employee. Not every opportunity will be a good match for you or the employer, and that is okay. Understanding the components of a good match will be the key to long term success. By marketing yourself, you will have a sound understanding of what positions will be a good match for you personally.

There are several components of marketing yourself that should be addressed, including your value and values, your integrity, your skills, and your needs. Before looking for a job, it would be worthwhile to write out each category. This exercise will help you to ask potential employers the right questions, which will assist in your own determination. Then practice with a friend. Remember, you are interviewing the employer as much as the employer is interviewing you.

Values are defined as "the abstract concepts of what is right, worthwhile or desirable; principles or standards."[9] Ask questions about the business's philosophies and goals (businesses should have both financial and nonfinancial goals). Specifically ask about patient care philosophies. Then discuss those values with which you can identify. Important values to you may include being on time, following company protocol, providing quality care of clients, or even volunteering at the local women's shelter. Think twice about taking a position where your values differ from those of the clinic or employer.

Under the subject of *your value,* you will want to itemize specifics such as the location of your primary education. Some schools have more prestige than others; build on this if it is possible. Include a list of your advanced education, including college (name, location, and degree), advanced aesthetic education classes (with whom and where). And, finally, include experience in the field in which you are looking to be employed.

Integrity is different from values. Integrity is defined as "uncompromising adherence to moral and ethical principles; *honesty*."[10] In this category you will want to ask questions about patient care, such as how complications are handled, how unhappy patients are handled, and how fee disputes are managed. Also, ask direct questions about the ethical principles of the company. There should be a written philosophy. Usually it is in the **Mission Statement**. Then consider if these ethical principles are similar to or the same as your own. They should be.

Your skills are important to an employer, but sometimes the position is not exactly what you are looking for. You may be underqualified or overqualified. You need to assess this with the employer. Ask questions about the specific skills needed and respond with information about your skills. If you are underqualified but there is otherwise a match, what training will be available to help you become qualified? How quickly will that happen and who will do the training? Will there be a pay raise once the training is complete? These are important questions to ask prior to committing to a position. What you hear at the interview and what comes to pass in a job are not always the same thing. It is in your best interest to put into writing some of what would otherwise be a "handshake" deal. This approach eliminates any future misunderstandings or hard feelings. If the employer is unwilling to do this, maybe it is not a match.

Your needs are especially important, but not exclusive of the employer's needs. The best situation is when you find a "need match." List your needs, such as salary (pay rate, pay schedule, and commission), benefits, vacation time, sick day policies, hours to be worked, desired job description, and any other important needs you may have. In advance, decide which ones you can compromise on and which ones will be a "deal breaker." Making this decision in advance prevents you from feeling "sour grapes" if you give in and then are regretful later on.

Once you have your credentials, your resume, and your marketing plan, you are ready to go get the job for which you are uniquely qualified.

Mission Statement
a clearly stated objective of a company to describe its goals

The clinician must be properly licensed by the state he or she plans to be working in.

Licensure and Insurance

The aesthetician must be licensed in the state where he or she plans to work. Confirmation of licensure should be provided to the employer and kept in the employee record. Many clinicians like to keep their license hanging in their treatment rooms for all to see. In some states, this is a requirement.

There are several types of insurance necessary for a spa business. For the aesthetician, the most important insurance policy will be the malpractice policy. This is the insurance policy that covers your actions when treating clients. If something goes wrong, this is the policy that will protect you. For you, as the individual aesthetician, getting proper coverage is a fact-finding mission. First, speak with your employer and find out what the status of coverage for your position will be. Second, find a reputable company and have a consultation with one of the agents. Take their counsel and then consider a discussion with an attorney to ensure your best interests are evaluated.

Liability Issues for the Clinician

Liability issues for the clinician are an important factor in preparing for a career. Our United States society is far more litigious than ever before. If something goes wrong, the client may be looking for someone to blame. Whether a case ever comes to settlement or trial, the stress of being blamed will be unbelievable, and it is a situation no clinician should be caught in.

There are many potential liability risks for aestheticians. The most common injuries at risk for lawsuits are scarring, burns, product reactions and allergies, and infections. Infection is most commonly the result of a clinician's failure to provide an adequate standard of care. Infections can happen in a variety of ways: failure to properly clean and sterilize implements including extractors, makeup brushes, electrodes, tweezers, bowls, reusable masks, or basically anything that touches the skin. Failure to wear gloves during treatments or a lack of understanding about the sterilization and contamination process can also lead to infections. The transmission of hepatitis C, **HIV/AIDS**, and **herpes simplex** should all be a concern to the aesthetician. Burns are unusual but can occur through the use of paraffin or electric blankets. The aesthetician must be alert to the potential for burns, checking in with the client about temperatures and removing the offending product if necessary. Product reactions including allergies are not uncommon. It is important for the aesthetician to listen to the client and be respectful if a previous allergy or sensitivity has occurred. Disregarding a client's history could create a product allergy and sensitivity that could be followed by an unpleasant conversation of "I told you so."

HIV/AIDS
acquired human immunodeficiency syndrome (AIDS) is caused by the human immunodeficiency virus (HIV)

herpes simplex
an infection caused by the herpes simplex virus, indicated by painful fluid-filled blisters on the skin and mucous membranes

Regulatory Agencies

The agencies that regulate the spas are not federalized, but implemented on a state by state basis. Therefore, it will be important for you to check with the licensing agency in your state to determine if there are any specific requirements related to your job, aside from general licensure.

Professional Organizations

Because our industry is so fractured, many organizations trying to accomplish lofty goals for our industry are in conflict with another organization with the same goals. It will be important over the coming years for us to support organizations that have our best interests in mind as we work toward goals to create uniform educational requirements.

Conclusion

The spa industry is one of the fastest growing business sectors in America. There are many types of spas and as such many opportunities —each with its own reward. Employees should be professional, educated, and willing to work hard to build their clientele. As treatments have become more sophisticated and our tools have become more advanced, we have the opportunity to provide our clients the treatments that may help to reduce the stress of an extraordinarily busy world. However, attention to training is required. Aestheticians should seek ongoing education to keep abreast of the latest technologies and options that are available for delivering quality services and treatments to clients. A spa experience should focus on meeting luxury and high standards while ensuring client comfort and safety requirements are met.

▶ ⟩ ⟩ TOP 10 TIPS TO TAKE TO THE CLINIC

1. Practice proper infection control.
2. Seek continuing education to stay abreast of changing treatments and technology.
3. Develop in-house training protocols to create consistency in treatments.
4. Keep the facility clean.
5. Follow OSHA regulations.
6. Conduct regular safety checks.
7. Conduct yourself with integrity.
8. Strive to offer high quality services.
9. Ensure that liability insurance is in place.
10. Create a career plan that meets your goals.

CHAPTER QUESTIONS

1. Name some examples of where the word "spa" may have originated.
2. What were the primary treatments offered in early spas?
3. What type of disinfectant is most effective for infection control?
4. Why is it important to follow OSHA guidelines?
5. What is the Bloodborne Pathogens Act?
6. What is the difference between disinfection and sterilization?
7. Why is it important to conduct water testing in a spa pool?
8. Why is continuing education important?
9. Why is a good employment match important?

CHAPTER REFERENCES

1. Bergel, R., & Leavy, H. (2003). *The Spa Encyclopedia*. Clifton Park, NY: Thomson Delmar Learning.
2. http://www.census.gov; http://www.dol.gov
3. D'Angelo, J., Dean, P., Deitz, S., Hinds, C., Lees, M., Miller, E., et al. (2003). *Milady's Standard Comprehensive Training for Estheticians*. Clifton Park, NY: Thomson Delmar Learning.
4. http://www.osha.gov
5. http://www.dca.ca.gov
6. http://www.dca.ca.gov
7. Elko, L., Rosenbach, K., & Sinnitt, J. (2003). Cutaneous Manifestations of Waterborne Infections. *Current Infectious Disease Reports* (5), 398–406; Current Science, Inc.
8. Elko, L., Rosenbach, K., & Sinnitt, J. (2003). Cutaneous Manifestations of Waterborne Infections. *Current Infectious Disease Reports* (5), 398–406; Current Science, Inc.
9. *Webster's College Dictionary*. (1992). New York: Random House (p. 1473).
10. *Webster's College Dictionary*. (1992). New York: Random House (p. 700).

Anatomy and Physiology of the Skin

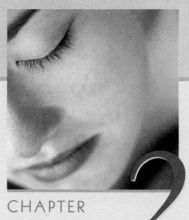

CHAPTER

2

After completing this chapter, you should be able to:

1. Know the layers of the skin.
2. Discuss and define the importance of melanocytes, keratinocytes, and fibroblasts.
3. Understand the importance of GAGs (glycosaminoglycans).
4. Describe the difference between intrinsic and extrinsic aging.
5. Describe transepidermal water loss (TEWL).
6. Understand the constituents of natural moisturizing factor (NMF).

"The beauty of a face is a frail ornament, a passing flower, a moment's brightness belonging only to the skin."[1] The skin is the largest human organ. It is our protection from outside elements, it identifies us, and it defines our beauty.

As clinicians in the field of dermal techniques, it is important for us to be familiar with the skin, its layers, and the cells within them. Your deeper understanding of skin structure and function will help you to be a better clinician. In turn, this will provide your client with improved results and safer care.

integumentary system (integument) the skin and its appendages (nails, hair, and sweat and oil glands)

INTRODUCTION

The skin and its appendages—nails, hair, nerve endings, sweat glands, and oil glands—compose the **integumentary system**, sometimes referred to as "integument." Skin not only keeps our bodies and its various components intact, but it is also, and equally important, our most immediate contact with our environment. Our skin senses vital information about the world in which we live, and, therefore, it ensures our survival.

While seemingly uniform and simple in its presentation and purpose, it is far more complex and variant than meets the eye. Skin varies in thickness and in sensitivity as well. Parts of it develop from brain tissues and remain attached to the brain through nerves, which conduct pleasure as well as pain.[2] These signals are vital to our success as a species. While not all of the sensations we feel are pleasurable, they all are purposeful. If we could not sense cold air, we would all freeze to death. If we could not feel a cut, we could bleed to death or die from infection. These sensations are detected by nerves, which in turn send the information to our brains for processing and translation. The skin overall possesses most of the nerve endings that transmit vital information about our environment to the brain. There are relatively few on our posterior sides; however, in lips, fingers, and genitals they are abundant.

Similarly, because the skin is our outermost organ, it also serves as a unique identifier, which we see and use to associate and differentiate one person from the next. Being the psychosocial creatures we are, we have put great emphasis on how others perceive the way we appear. The way we dress, decorate, and posture ourselves conveys gender, age, strength, and, most noticeably, attractiveness.

The appearance of the skin has become an indicator of beauty in our society, and we strive to optimize it. New scientific developments promise creams that act longer, stronger, or faster to help one appear younger. Some consumers are extraordinarily sophisticated in finding the newest treatments and the latest products to counteract the aging process. Others are overwhelmed by the options available to them. Either way, there are things we can do to maintain and even regain beautiful skin. In order to do so we must ask ourselves, how do we determine what works best and why? How much change is even possible? Even the savviest of consumers need help answering these questions. Most of them will turn to you for advice. It is here our quest begins. (See Table 2–1.)

So why do we need to know about skin anatomy and physiology? As an aesthetician performing body treatments, the skin, muscles, and cardiovascular system are your media. It is important to understand the skin, its functions, and its potential responses to avoid injuries such as burns. Furthermore, certain body treatments can cause dehydration, and an understanding of the skin will help to head off any potential problems as well. (See Figure 2–1.)

Table 2–1   Fun Facts About the Skin
***Fun Facts About the Skin*[3]**
Humans shed millions of dead skin flakes every minute.
In adults, the skin usually covers about two square meters (about the size of a shower curtain) and weighs about 7 pounds. It also has 300 million skin cells.
The skin is between 1.5 mm and 4 mm thick, about as thick as a few sheets of paper.
The thickest areas of the skin (plantar and palmar regions) contain no hair follicles or sweat glands.
Millions of coiled sweat glands discharge sweat and salts to the surface, where evaporation begins to cool the body in seconds.
Just below the surface, the dermis feeds miles of blood vessels with nutrients.
The brain and skin become connected very early in fetal development. Even in the womb, a baby's hand can feel its way to the mouth.
Touch is the first sense to develop.
The skin's array of nerves is sensitive enough to feel the weight of a mosquito as it lands.
On average, each square inch of skin contains 10 hairs, 15 sebaceous glands, 100 sweat glands, and 3.2 feet of blood vessels.

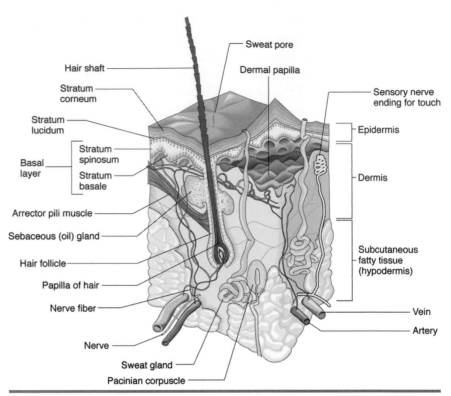

Figure 2–1 The skin may be simple in its presentation and purpose, but it is far more complex than meets the eye

An active organ, the skin provides protection, conveys sensation, sends signals, regulates temperature, produces vitamin D3, and helps rid our bodies of unneeded or threatening components.[4] It is elastic–it stretches when we frown or smile or bend, and regains its normality when we relax.[5]

SKIN PHYSIOLOGY

As we have already discussed, skin does so much more than just hold the other organs in place.

Not much thicker than a sheet of paper, skin is quite complex. In general terms, it protects, senses, and aids temperature regulation, excretion, immunologic responses, and metabolism.

Protection

Protection is one of the skin's main functions. Skin acts as a barrier against intruders such as water, ultraviolet light, bacteria, and fungi, as well as against minor trauma. The skin is a mostly waterproof sheath that protects against too much moisture entering or escaping from within.

It also secretes acids that could otherwise allow bacteria and viruses to penetrate the skin and cause disease, or even death.[6] Likewise, the skin acts as armor against foreign matter. While a cut does hurt, it is preferable to that same cut causing trauma to an internal organ. The final way the skin protects us is against the damaging effects of solar rays. The pigment melanin is produced as an active response to ultraviolet light, thus preventing cellular damage. This will be discussed in more detail later in this chapter.

Sensation and Communication

Skin is capable of receiving a diverse amount of tactile information from a variety of receptors. Neural receptors, some of them quite elaborate, mediate touch, position, pressure, temperature, and pain. The communication goes two ways and occurs instinctively. The skin releases signals such as blushing, **pheromones** (unique chemical signals), and body odor.

> **pheromones**
> chemical substances, the release of which may affect the behavior or physiology of a recipient

   The four senses recognized by the skin are touch (pressure being sustained by contact), cold, heat, and pain.[7] Nerves that receive and send these sensory signals to the brain show a variety of sensory endings, including expanded tips (Merkel's disks and Ruffini endings), encapsulated endings (Pacinian corpuscles, Meissner's corpuscles, and Krause's end bulbs), and simple naked nerve endings. Many sensory nerves terminate around hair follicles. Expanded or encapsulated nerve endings can occur also in areas of the body removed from the skin, explaining "deep" pain we can feel, such as from a kidney punch.

Thermoregulation

Skin is critical for regulating body temperature.[8] The body's optimal internal, or core, temperature is maintained by actions of blood vessels in the lower layer of the skin. Blood vessels will insulate the body's core temperature from both internal and external temperature variations by constricting and relaxing blood flow. When we are exposed to cold, blood vessels in the lower layer of the skin constrict. This allows the blood to bypass that which would cool it as the skin cools to the outside temperature. When it is warm, those blood vessels dilate and heat is radiated outward. Perspiration evaporates off the surface of the skin and cools us. To this effect, body heat is conserved.

   Although normal core body temperature is 37° Celsius or 98.6° Fahrenheit, skin surface is normally cooler, around 33° Celsius or 91° Fahrenheit.[9] The surface temperature of the skin depends on the temperature of the air that touches it and the amount of time spent in that air. Weather factors such as wind and humidity affect skin temperature, and temperature at different points of the skin surface can differ dramatically. After exertions on a windy and snowy day, one climber on Denali reported the temperature of his big toe to be 42° Fahrenheit at the same time that the surface of his chest measured 88° Fahrenheit.[10]

Metabolism

Blood vessels within the lower layer of the skin also provide nutrition for the skin. Blood flow carries some of the minerals and vitamins that are critical for skin's health and appearance, such as oxygen. Oxygen requirements for skin are *greater* than that of connective tissue, and if not enough oxygen is supplied, the health of the skin may suffer. This is why smoking cigarettes may cause problems with healing. Skin health affects not only how we look, but also how quickly and smoothly cat scratches and paper cuts heal.

Immunologic Response

Skin contains specialized cells to protect it and the body within. **Mast cells** and **Langerhans' cells** defend the skin against microorganisms. Langerhans cells detect antigens in the uppermost layer of the skin. Mast cells are poised to create an inflammatory response should the skin be injured.[11] This is evidenced by allergic reactions. Mast cells are responsible for **histamine** and related responses to mosquito bites and bee stings. (See Figures 2–2 and 2–3.)

Excretion

Through the sweat glands the skin releases fluid and toxins. These same glands are important regulators of body temperature as mentioned above.[12]

■ SKIN ANATOMY

If one of the skin's main functions is to act as a barrier against intruding substances, how, then, do lotions that we apply "soak in"? The primary answer is the **appendages**.

Appendages are defined as smaller parts to a greater part. For the skin, they include the pilosebaceous unit (hair follicle and accompanying **sebaceous glands** and **arrector pili muscle**), sweat glands, and nails.[13] Appendages originate in the uppermost layer of the skin (the epidermis), but extend in pockets of epidermis into the lower layer, the dermis.

External substances such as skin creams, ointments, and salves can enter the skin through the appendages of the hair and sweat glands (see Figure 2–4), or through the intercellular spaces between

mast cells
large tissue cells present in the skin that produce histamine and other acute symptoms of allergic reactions

Langerhans' cells
cells intimately involved in the immune response of the skin

histamine
an amino acid histidine, found in the body

appendages
any anatomical structures associated with a larger structure; the skin's appendages include hair, glands, and pores

sebaceous glands
small glands usually located next to the hair follicle in the dermis that release fatty liquids onto the hair follicle to soften hair and skin

arrector pili muscle
an involuntary muscle arising out of the skin; causes goose bumps

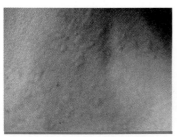

Figure 2–2 The skin contains specialized cells to protect it

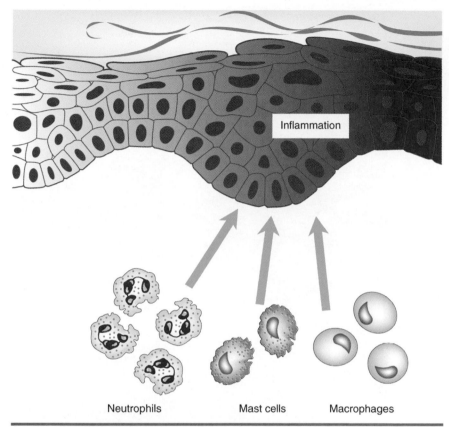

Neutrophils   Mast cells   Macrophages

Figure 2–3 Mast cells and Langerhans' cells defend the skin against microorganisms

the **cornified** cells; smaller molecules can pass through cells at the surface of the skin.

Sweat Glands

You can think of sweat glands as simple tubes. They are vital for regulating body temperature. Because of the composition of what they carry to the surface, sweat glands also influence water balance and ions.

Ordinary **eccrine sweat glands** are located over most of the body, and large **apocrine sweat glands** are concentrated in axillary (underarm), pubic, and perianal areas,[14] which develop at puberty.[15] Although sweat from the apocrine glands is initially odorless, it can mix with bacteria on the skin and acquire an odor.

Normal, healthy adults secrete about one pint of sweat per day, and more with physical activity.[16] Because of daily loss of water, everyone needs to actively replace water lost inside the body, regardless of the individual's activity level. The more active a person is, the more water needs

cornified
hardening or thickening of the skin

apocrine sweat glands
larger of the sweat glands, which are housed in axillary (under the arm), pubic, and perianal areas

eccrine sweat glands
smaller of the sweat glands, which reside all over the body

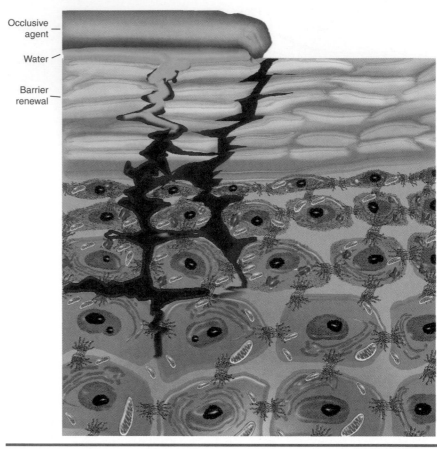

Occlusive agent

Water

Barrier renewal

Figure 2–4 Creams, ointments, and salves enter the skin through the appendages and through the intercellular spaces between the cornified cells. Smaller molecules can pass through cells at the surface of the skin.

The skin's appendages (see Figure 2–5) are important in healing, especially superficial healing and protection of the skin. When the skin is superficially injured over a limited surface, it can grow back quickly because of epithelial cells remaining in deeper hair follicles and sweat glands. This is important to understand when we begin to discuss wound healing and our care of the client after aggressive treatments.

to be replaced. As much as four cups of water can be lost during hard exercise. In order to avoid dehydration, water should be consumed regularly throughout the day and more before, during, and after exercise. When a person has become thirsty, he or she is already dehydrated, so it is important to consume fluids regardless of thirst. Symptoms of dehydration include dizziness, disorientation, and clumsiness.[17]

Hair Follicles

Hair is a type of modified skin. It grows everywhere on a person's body except the palmar and plantar regions of hands and feet. Hair is the densest on the head, neck, and shoulder regions, where there can be 300 to 900 per cm^2. Conversely, there are about 100 per cm^2 on the torso and limbs.[18] Hair follicles are tubular. They protrude deep into the skin to develop and nourish the hair. The hair follicle contains epidermal cells

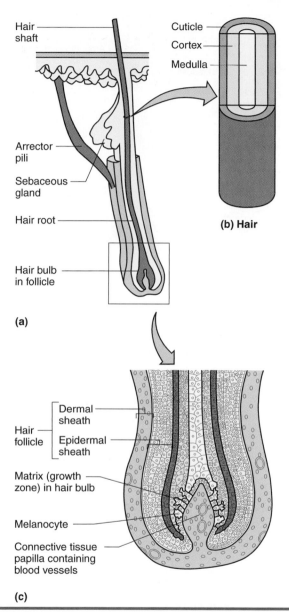

Figure 2–5 The skin's appendages, which include the sebaceous glands and arrector pili muscle, sweat glands, and nails, are important in healing, especially superficial wounds

while the hair itself is **keratin**. Hair follicles have several distinct anatomic components including *the bulb, the root,* and *the papilla.*

The hair follicle, gland, nerve, and muscle are called the **pilosebaceous unit**. Hair follicles are associated with sebaceous glands (small masses of cells and fat associated with hair follicles) that lubricate the hair; nerve endings that detect motion of the hair shaft and control

keratin
protein cell found in the skin, hair, and nails; insoluble in water, weak acids, or alkalis

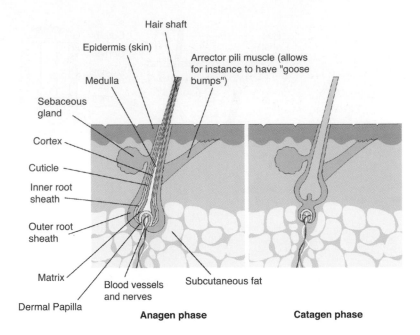

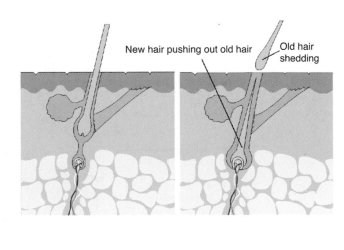

Figure 2–6 Hair growth is a complex process

pilosebaceous unit
hair follicle and accompanying sebaceous glands and arrector pili muscles

anagen phase
hair growth phase in which growth is actually occurring

catagen phase
intermediate stage in the hair growth phase

telogen phase
stage of hair growth during which the hair is at rest

piloerection ("goose bumps"); and smooth muscle, which actually creates the "goose bumps."[19] The sebaceous glands that are most active reside on the face, chest, and back.

All hair goes through an **anagen phase** (growth), a **catagen phase** (transitional), and a **telogen phase** (resting) (see Figure 2–6)—the hair grows, resides for a while, and then falls out.[20] This growth cycle varies in different parts of the body. For instance, the entire cycle takes four months for eyelashes and three to four years for scalp hair.

As we will see, this process of division, growth, and maturation somewhat resembles that of the skin's top layer. In both cases cells go through a process of hardening and then "sloughing," or being shed. But when cells at the bottom of the hair follicle **slough**, they create a column of keratinized (hardened, "horny") cells. This is the hair that grows up through the shaft and extends through the follicle. Hair growth is a complex process, but understanding this process is key to the success of hair removal with lasers or light. Lasers are known to be effective only on hairs in the growth (anagen) phase.

Nails

Like hair, nails are also a type of modified skin.[21] They are formed from hardened cells in the top layer of skin.

Nails of the fingers and toes protect their sensitive tips. They provide support for the tips of our digits and assist in picking up objects. While effective, they are not necessary for living, and neither are details of their histology necessary for us to know.

■ LAYERS OF THE SKIN

The skin comprises two main layers, the top (epidermis) (see Figure 2–7), which is tough and, because of its exposure, constantly being worn down and replaced.[22] It contains no blood vessels or nerves and is vital

slough
cast-off skin, feathers, hair, or horn

hypodermis
layer of subcutaneous fat and connective tissue lying beneath the epidermis

The outermost layer of the skin is the epidermis. It shields us from the environment, potential injury, bacteria, pollution, and almost everything else that wants to get in. The lower layer of the skin, called the dermis, is the support, providing the epidermis with strength and stability.

Beneath the dermis is subcutaneous fat (**hypodermis**), a thermal barrier and mechanical cushion that varies in thickness from person to person and at different places on the body. Sturdy collagen within the hypodermis prevents tearing and sustains the main dermal strength.

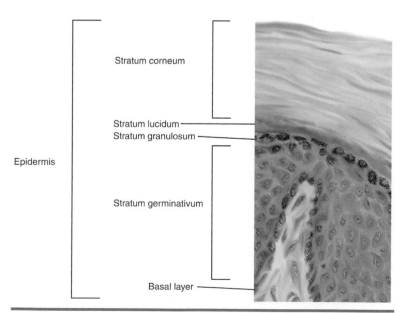

Stratum corneum

Stratum lucidum
Stratum granulosum

Epidermis

Stratum germinativum

Basal layer

Figure 2–7 The epidermis contains no blood vessels or nerves and is vital in preventing loss of moisture from the body

dermis
the second layer of skin, which is
responsible for attaching the skin to
the body

subcutaneous
beneath the skin

epidermis
outermost, avascular, protective layer
of skin

avascular
lacking in blood vessels and, thus,
having a poor blood supply

keratinocyte
any cell in the skin, hair, or nails that
produces keratin

stratum lucidum
sublayer of the epidermis characterized
by the appearance of granules and the
disappearance of the nucleus within the
skin cells

stratum spinosum
sublayer of the epidermis intertwined
with desmosomes

stratum basale
the lowest layer of the epidermis. The
statum basale (basal layer) houses
germinal cells and regenerating cells
for all layers of the epidermis.

psoriasis
a chronic skin disease characterized by
inflammation and white scaly patches

in preventing loss of moisture from the body. The deeper layer of the skin (**dermis**) and the **subcutaneous** (meaning "beneath" the skin) fat beneath it lend strength and elasticity to the skin. Within both layers of skin are sublayers with cells that perform specific functions.

If you look at a microscopic slice of skin, it will look as though some objects, such as hair follicles, project from the dermis through the epidermis. This is not really the case. The epidermis encases these objects and projects down into the dermis beneath it.

Let us drill down into the skin from above.

The Epidermis

The **epidermis** is the top layer, the outer skin, the skin that we see. It contains tiny pockets that house sweat glands and pilosebaceous glands.[23] Compared to the dermis beneath the epidermis, it is often very thin, approximately 0.12 mm, but its thickness also varies dramatically over the body.[24] It is thickest on the palms of the hands and soles of the feet and thinnest on the eyelids.

The epidermis is **avascular** (without blood vessels), impermeable to water, physically tough, and dry at the surface to impede the growth of microorganisms. It is continually replacing itself. When the epidermis is injured or diseased, its replacement speeds up in response, and this is important to us as clinicians. In short, it is our self-replicating defense against everything outside of us.

Unlike other cellular components of the body, such as nerves, epidermal cells are born and die and are replaced by new ones. If all of the cells of the body behaved like those of the epidermis, there would be no spinal cord paralysis or diabetes because cellular renewal would heal those injuries and diseases.

Within the epidermis are five less distinct "sublayers." These sublayers are not composed of different cell *types*, but rather differ more because they reflect *stages* of hardening, maturation, and eventual death in the migration of their major cell type, the **keratinocyte**.[25]

The "sublayers" of the epidermis include, from the top, the stratum corneum, the **stratum lucidum**, the stratum granulosum, the **stratum spinosum**, and the **stratum basale**.

The Stratum Corneum

The stratum corneum is the "top" or superficial layer of the epidermis. It varies in thickness: Thin on the upper arm, it is thick on the soles of the feet, palms of the hands, and other areas of chronic friction. Its thickness can be affected by simple dry skin as well as by disease processes such as **psoriasis**.

Each month the cells of the basal layer (bottom layer of the epidermis) make their way through the layers of the epidermis into the stratum corneum. The cells begin as healthy plump cells with a fully functioning nucleus. But as they near the summit, they shrivel and flatten out.[26] The cells completed their gradual transition to death and are soon to be sloughed off, but this is what makes them protective. It is actually this layer that is "polished" by microdermabrasion.

Although it is drier than lower skin layers, the stratum corneum contains a compound, the **natural moisturizing factor (NMF)**. NMF helps to keep the skin soft and moisturized even in dry climates.[27] NMF is composed of **amino acids** and filaggrin, water-soluble chemicals capable of absorbing large quantities of water. The presence of NMF in the stratum corneum is critical for soft and flexible skin. Although NMF is contained only in the uppermost layer of the skin, its existence is made possible by ingredients provided by deeper structures.[28]

Natural moisturizing factor gives the cells of the stratum corneum their ability to bind with water. NMF is found only in the stratum corneum, and it is solely responsible for the regulation of water in the very superficial layers of the stratum corneum. Not surprisingly, its presence is diminished by age and excessive exposure to soap. This is key to understanding the phenomenon of dry skin.

It is worth noting that NMF and TEWL have nothing to do with water loss associated with sweating. It is a common misconception that drinking water will improve hydration levels of the skin. This is simply not true. Drinking water improves water level inside the body, but is used up there. The best way to rehydrate the skin is by applying a topical moisturizer.

The Stratum Lucidum

This thin, clear band ("lucidum" means clear or bright) of closely packed cells is most prominent in areas of thick skin and may be absent in other areas.[30]

The Stratum Granulosum

Like the other sublayers of the epidermis, this layer signals transition of the cells within it.[31] It is in this layer that the keratin loses the nucleus and **organelles**, becoming flat, before moving farther up into the stratum corneum. It is called the stratum granulosum because of the granules that now appear in the cells. In effect, these granules write the death warrant of the cell, for as the granules grow in size, the nucleus—the power generator of the cell—disintegrates and dies.[32]

Psoriasis is a genetic malfunction of the epidermal cellular reproduction rate. The accelerated process creates a phenomenon known as psoriasis plaques. Psoriasis can also be environmentally precipitated, but usually people are genetically predisposed.

As long as we are not submerged, our bodies constantly lose water via evaporation through our skin. This gentle process is called **transepidermal water loss (TEWL)**,[29] and we are totally unaware of it. In normal epidermis the water content decreases the closer we get to the surface. Water makes up to 70 to 75 percent of the weight of layers beneath, but only 10 to 15 percent of the weight of the stratum corneum. When too much water evaporates, not only our skin but also our bodies suffer ill effects. Preventing excessive water loss is important both to the skin itself and to the body as a whole.

transepidermal water loss (TEWL)
the process by which our bodies constantly lose water via evaporation

Within the granular layer is a compound called **filaggrin**. Filaggrin assists keratinocytes in creating the natural moisturizing factor found in the stratum corneum. Filaggrin also combines with other cells found within the granular layer to create strength and stability for the epidermis.

natural moisturizing factor (NMF)
compound found only in the top layer of the skin, which gives cells their ability to bind with water

amino acids
organic compound that contains an amino group and a carboxylic group

organelles
a specific location within the cell

The Stratum Spinosum

Stratum spinosum means "spiny layer." Cells in this sublayer are intertwined with tiny structures called **desmosomes**. Under the microscope desmosomes resemble hair combed with an eggbeater, which is why this part is often called the "prickly cell" layer. The hair-like desmosomes permit materials to move around them in the intercellular space (the spaces between cells). **Lamellar granules** are also found here. These granules control lipids that migrate to the stratum corneum and become another component of "natural moisturizing factor."

In this, the first leg of the journey, keratinocytes depart the basal layer and show the first signs of **keratinization**. Here also we find lamellar granules, organelles that deliver fats to the stratum corneum. These granules contain the **lipids** and other components such as cholesterol, fatty acids, **ceramides**, and enzymes necessary to produce the *natural moisturizing factor*. Once these granules reach the stratum corneum, they release their contents and cause the natural moisturizing factor to occur.

The Stratum Basale

The basement of the epidermis is appropriately called the "basal layer." It anchors the epidermis to the dermis. This layer contains germinal cells, cells of regeneration, for all sublayers of the epidermis. It is here that stem cells produce two types of cells. Basal cells remain in the basal layer, creating a solid skin foundation, and keratinocytes begin their upward migration to the stratum corneum.

Special Epidermal Cells   Within the epidermis there are four types of specialized cells: the keratinocytes, melanocytes, Langerhans' cells, and Merkel cells. (See Table 2–2.)

Table 2–2   Specialized Epidermal Cells

Specialized Epidermal Cells	Location	Function
Keratinocytes	Generated in the strata basale, and half begin to migrate upward, eventually to be sloughed off	Basic skin cells that collectively make up the skin; undergo desquamation
Melanocytes	Between the epidermis and the dermis	Secrete pigments that give skin, hair, and eyes their color
Langerhans' cells	In the strata spinosum and strata basale	Patrol the epidermis for foreign invaders, ingest them, for removal by the lymphatic system
Merkel cells	By nerve endings throughout epidermis	Exact function unclear; likely involved in sensation

Keratinocytes   The majority of cells in the epidermis are keratinocytes, cells generated in its lower or basal sublayer but destined, half the time, to depart. Fifty percent of the keratinocytes produced remain in the basal sublayer of the epidermis (and are then, as you saw above, identified as basal cells). The others, retaining their keratinocyte identity and a certain apparent ambition, begin moving up, passing through the remaining sublayers to the surface, becoming hard and cornified, and finally being sloughed off.[33]

During differentiation, keratinocytes go through critical changes. The shape flattens, then organelles are "lost" and fibrous proteins are shaped, and, finally, as the cell becomes dehydrated, the cell membrane thickens.

The process of moving from the basal layer to the stratum corneum and then sloughing off is called "**desquamation** or differentiation." It takes approximately 28 to 35 days in younger people and up to 45 days as we age, and when it takes longer, it shows in the appearance of the skin. Delays in the migration process as well as extrinsic factors such as smoking, solar damage, and pollution cause our skin to turn sallow and gray. It causes the complaint so often heard from our clients, that "my skin just looks dull and dirty."

Melanocytes   Located in or near the basal layer, **melanocytes** (see Figures 2–8 and 2–9) occupy the junction between the epidermis and the dermis. They secrete the pigment, **melanin**, that lends color to skin, eyes, and hair. Melanin protects the skin from ultraviolet light and is produced in response to it. Melanin is also produced in response to genetic and hormonal cues.

After melanocytes have produced melanin, they transfer it to keratinocytes via small appendages that act like eyedroppers. Regardless of whether they carry cargo, keratinocytes continue their migration toward the surface.[34] In this cellular relationship *melanocytes* are the melanin-*making* cells and keratinocytes are the melanin-*taking* cells, and thus it is that, although melanocytes produce melanin, in the end keratinocytes contain it. The proportion of melanocytes to keratinocytes varies from 1:4 to 1:10, with melanocyte proportion decreasing with age. As we age, therefore, our ability to protect our skin with melanin decreases.

Both injury and inflammation can cause increases in melanin production. Such an injury is known as **postinflammatory hyperpigmentation** and is a recognized complication of both microdermabrasion and peeling. Pigmentation in both its overproduction and underproduction forms will be discussed below.

Langerhans' Cells   Found in the lower layers of the epidermis, Langerhans' cells engage in surveillance against would-be intruders.[35] Although

---

The basal layer houses several types of basal cells, including **stem cells**, amplifying cells, and **postmitotic cells**. In part the stratum basale creates its own stability, and in part it commences the cell migration and maturation toward the more superficial layers. The cells of the basal layer form the "basement" of the epidermis, attaching to the dermis below and the spiny layer above. This is the layer that generates the epidermal cellular process.

desmosomes
small hair-like structures in the spiny layer (stratum spinosum) of the epidermis

lamellar granules
control lipids that produce NMF

keratinization
a progressive maturation of the keratin cell in the movement through the stratum corneum

lipids
fat or fat-like substances, descriptive not chemical

filaggrin
synthesizes lipids (fats) that are thought to serve as "intercellular cement"; important component of NMF

ceramides
a class of lipids that does not contain glycerol

The relative number of melanocytes is the same for men and women and indeed for all races. The major contribution to the depth of skin color is melanocyte *activity* rather than quantity. While melanocytes partially protect the skin from UV radiation, the clinician should never assume that those who tan easily or have darker skin types are protected from skin cancers.

postmitotic cells
cells that have completed mitotic division

stem cells
unspecialized cell that gives rise to a specific specialized cell

desquamation
shedding of cells, such as at the stratum corneum

melanocytes
type of cell (in the epidermis) that produces the pigment melanin

melanin
pigment that protects skin from ultraviolet damage

postinflammatory hyperpigmentation
hyperpigmentation that occurs after injury to the skin

Merkel cells
usually close to nerve endings and may be involved in sensory perception

Light skin

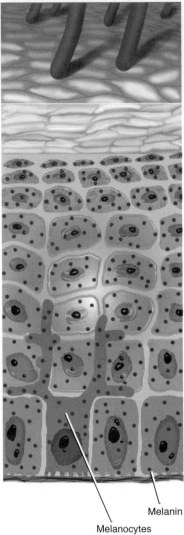

Melanin

Melanocytes

Figure 2–8 Melanocytes secrete melanin that lends color to skin, eyes, and hair

smaller in breadth than keratinocytes, they stretch finger-like probes between keratinocytes to the surface, where they scan like periscopes. Upon encountering "bad bacteria" they "acquire" them and transport the offenders to T lymphocytes in the regional lymph nodes for disposal.

Merkel Cells   **Merkel cells** are associated with the nerve endings found in the epidermis. Their specific function remains unclear, but, as they are numerous about the lip, hard palate, palms, finger and foot pads, and proximal nail folds, they are likely involved in sensation.[36,37]

Dark skin

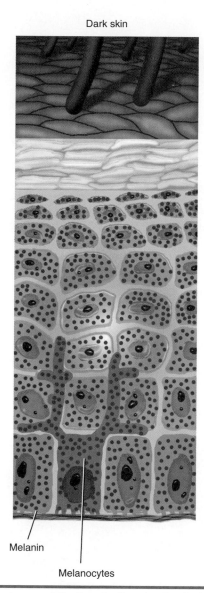

Melanin

Melanocytes

Figure 2–9 The major contribution to the depth of skin color is melanocyte *activity* rather than quantity

The Dermis

In our continued drilling into the skin we encounter the second, deeper layer of skin, the dermis. (See Figure 2–10.) The dermis provides the vital function of attaching skin to body. (See Figure 2–11.)

The dermis is crisscrossed with three types of fibers that lend strength and elasticity. These fibers—**reticulin, collagen,** and **elastin**—form a network that creates stability for the skin. Type I collagen runs

reticulin
a water soluble protein in the connective tissue framework of reticular tissue

collagen
a water soluble protein found in connective tissues. Particularly, type I collagen forms a network in the epidermis, and it is credited with providing skin with its tensile strength and firmness.

elastin
connective tissues

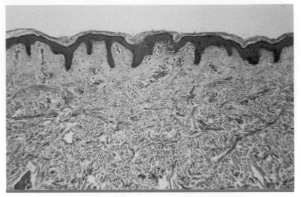

Figure 2-10 The dermal cells include fibro-blasts, ground substance, and mast cells

throughout the dermis and is responsible for its tensile strength and providing skin with its youthful appearance of tightness, firmness, and fullness.[38] The combined strength of these tissues anchors the epidermis above to the subcutaneous tissue below.

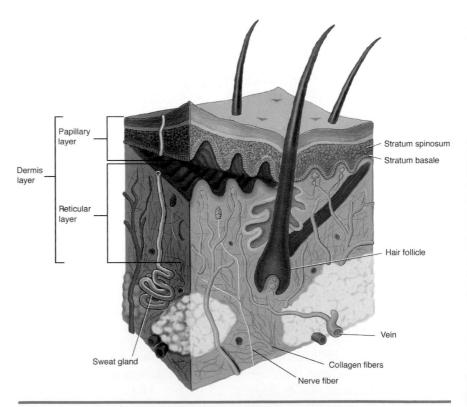

Figure 2-11 On its superficial side the dermis holds to the epidermis; on its distal side it attaches to subcutaneous tissue

Epidermal appendages such as sweat glands and hair follicles are embedded in the dermis, which also serves as the end point for blood vessels and nerves.[39]

The dermis, which varies but is about 2 mm thick, is further subdivided into the papillary and reticular layers.[40] This subdivision is based on differences in collagen texture.[41]

Papillary Dermis

Papillary dermis, the most superficial layer of the dermis, is the first skin layer to contain capillary blood vessels, small nerves, and lymphatic vessels.

Because the papillary dermis contains blood vessels and blood vessels provide temperature changes when they constrict or dilate, it is papillary dermis that is specifically responsible for thermoregulation of the body. When, in performing microdermabrasion, you encounter "pin-point" bleeding, you have arrived at the papillary dermis. Does that not increase your respect for the thickness of the epidermis?

In addition to its "holding" properties, the papillary dermis has another very important function in regulating the appearance of skin surface, for this sublayer houses **glycosaminoglycans (GAGs)**. GAGs are a variety of "chains" made of polysaccharide, a type of complex carbohydrate. Attracted almost fanatically to water, GAGs are thought capable of binding up to 1,000 times their weight in water.[45] Think for a moment about the padding this provides. This moisture-attracting property makes them one of the most important components in our study of the skin. Many histology studies of the skin show a decrease in the number of GAGs with age.[46]

Reticular Dermis

Reticular dermis is located beneath papillary dermis and rests on the thick pad of fat known as subcutaneous tissue. Here lies the real anchor of the skin.

Within the **reticular dermis** are structures called **rete-pegs**. These "pegs" extend up into the epidermis (and similar structures extend from above down into the dermis) to hold the dermis to the epidermis. These structures are responsible for holding the epidermis and dermis together to create "the skin." Capillary networks run through rete-pegs like tiny elevators, bringing nutrients to the epidermis. It is widened vessels in the rete-pegs that cause "broken capillaries." People with transparent or very light skin may flush or blush, causing a dilation of the capillaries in the rete-pegs.

On its superficial side the dermis holds the epidermis at the **dermal-epidermal junction** (DEJ). On its distal side it attaches to subcutaneous tissue.

Collagen in the papillary dermis is finely textured.[42] It contains projections, called **papillae**, that fit the dermis to the epidermis.[43] We are accustomed to using these uniquely individual ridged patterns in footprinting and fingerprinting.[44]

dermal-epidermal junction
(DEJ) superficial side of the dermis, connected to the epidermis by subcutaneous tissue

papillae
projections from dermis into epidermis that hold them together

glycosaminoglycans (GAGs)
polysaccharide chains, most prominent in the dermis, that bind with water, smoothing and softening the surface from below; most abundant GAG is hyaluronic acid

reticular dermis
sublayer of the dermis that connects the dermis to the epidermis and is home to the skin's appendages (nails, hair, glands)

The reticular dermis houses the appendages of the skin, nerves, and blood vessels. It is loaded with collagen, blood vessels, and nerve endings.

Collagen in this layer ("reticular" means "like a network") is larger and more coarsely textured.[48] In the example of a cow's skin after "tanning" it is the cow's dermis that makes the leather.[49]

rete-pegs
anatomic feature that holds the dermis and epidermis together

fibroblasts
cells that produce connective tissue

ground substance
consists mainly of glycosaminoglycans (hyaluronic acid, chondroitin sulfate, and dermatan sulfate); involved in maintenance and repair of dermis

urticaria pigmentosa
allergic reactions such as hives with a large number of mast cells

Special Dermal Cells   There are many specialized dermal cells. Their functions range from directing the production of collagen and ground substance to providing nutrients and removing waste from the skin. (See Table 2–3.)

Fibroblast Cells   **Fibroblasts** are the "command" cells for the dermis. They direct the production of collagen, elastin, *reticulin,* and the **ground substance** for the dermis. In response to injury, fibroblasts proliferate to manufacture new collagen, from which scarring occurs.[47]

Mast Cells   Along with lymphocytes and macrophages, the mast cell resides in connective tissue of the dermis, usually in the neighborhood of blood vessels. These cells protect against injury and invasion. Release of histamine by mast cells produces the inflammation that ousts intruders and begins wound healing.[50] In allergic reactions manifested in the skin, such as hives, there are large numbers of mast cells. Clinicians will see this in a condition such as **urticaria pigmentosa**.

Ground Substance   Through diffusion, ground substance provides nutrients to and removes wastes from other tissue components.[51] It is integral to the healing process. As a wound heals, the available ground substance creates a moister wound that will heal more quickly. It is constantly undergoing synthesis and degradation. The ground substance of the dermis consists largely of glycosaminoglycans. Age probably brings a decrease in the ground substance.

■ HYPODERMIS OR SUBCUTANEOUS TISSUE

Under the reticular dermis lies the hypodermis, or subcutaneous fat. (See Figure 2–12.) It is made up of clumps of fat-filled cells called **adipose cells**. It is the "cushion layer" of the skin and helps protect internal organs from blows, and it also acts as an insulator, conserving body heat.[52]

Table 2–3   Specialized Dermal Cells

Specialized Dermal Cells	Location	Function
Fibroblasts	Reticular Dermis, Papillary Dermis	Direct the production of collagen, reticulin, and ground substance
Mast Cells	Papillary Dermis	Protect skin against invasion and infection
Ground Substance	Reticular Dermis, Papillary Dermis	Provide nutrients and remove waste

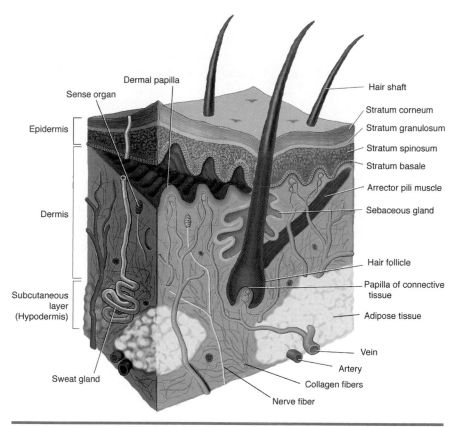

Epidermis

Dermis

Subcutaneous layer (Hypodermis)

Sense organ

Dermal papilla

Sweat gland

Hair shaft

Stratum corneum

Stratum granulosum

Stratum spinosum

Stratum basale

Arrector pili muscle

Sebaceous gland

Hair follicle

Papilla of connective tissue

Adipose tissue

Vein

Artery

Collagen fibers

Nerve fiber

Figure 2–12 The hypodermis is made up of clumps of fat-filled cells called adipose cells

The attachment of subcutaneous tissue to reticular dermis is not tight or rigid. Rather it is loose, allowing the skin a degree of shifting movement over muscle and skeletal structures. The subcutaneous tissue is crisscrossed with connective tissue to fibers and layers interspersed with fat to hold it together. When pockets of fat accumulate between the connective tissue bands beyond the ability of the connective tissue to hold it smooth, the appearance is called "cellulite or 'orange-peel' skin." Because women generally have thinner skin and less rigid connective tissue bands than men, "cellulite" is generally more apparent in women. It is also more likely to appear in certain areas of the body as well, such as the hips, thighs, and buttocks.

adipose cells
cells that contain stored fat in connective tissue

> Because women generally have thinner skin and less rigid connective tissue bands than men, "cellulite" is generally more apparent in women.

◾ SKIN HEALTH OVER TIME

As children, we take our soft, pliable, quickly healing integument for granted. We play outside, cavort in any available water, and roam hills, valleys, and flats. And during this time, our skin is absorbing the effects of this "trauma." The effects are not all bad, but they are certainly cumulative. Every bit of "exposure" has its consequences.

Realistically, we cannot completely avoid the sun. And we humans, at least a hefty majority of us, are idolaters of the sun. In an earlier time, people of wealth, good breeding, and leisure valued a pale, tanless complexion. It was in the late twentieth century that sun-bronzed skin took on its sexy aura of vigor and well-being. It connoted the ability to spend leisure time on beaches, golf courses, and tennis courts. Within boundaries, sun exposure is not all bad; in fact, we need the sun. Although we can get some vitamin D from plant and animal sources, sunlight on our skin is responsible for up to 90 percent of the vitamin D our bodies depend upon.[53] In tight conjunction with calcium, neither one of which works well without the other, vitamin D gives our bones tensile strength,[54] thus the reason for enriching milk with vitamin D.

Without question, however, many people get more sun exposure than is necessary for bone health. People who work outside are hard-pressed to avoid the effects of weather, even with generous applications of sunscreen. Even if the sun never touches us, we are bombarded with tiny molecular renegades (radiation) that do their damage. As long as we live, we cannot completely avoid damage to the skin, and it will age.

The aging process is both complex and yet simple. Simply put, it is the degradation of the dermis and epidermis over time that leaves the skin thin, lacking elasticity, lined and speckled with pigmentation. A reduction in **skin turgor** occurs.[55] Loss of adhesion between the layers of the epidermis as well as between the epidermis and dermis create a greater tendency for injury and more visible effects of gravity (wrinkles and folds). Decreases in filaggrin and the natural moisturizing factor mean dry and flaky skin. Wound healing slows from decrements in Langerhans' cells.[56]

To further understand the process of aging, we employ the terms **intrinsic aging** and **extrinsic aging**. Intrinsic aging occurs by virtue of genetics and gravity—it is unavoidable. Extrinsic aging is the portion for which we are responsible. It is aging attributable to external factors such as the sun, pollution, and smoking.

skin turgor
the flexibility of the skin

extrinsic aging
changes that are brought on by the effects of the environment and our choices relating to them, specifically sun exposure

intrinsic aging
changes that would occur over time without the effects of any environmental factors

Intrinsic Aging

Because genetics plays a noteworthy role in the aging process, part of its individual effects are out of our hands. The longer we live, the more likely we will face our mother or father in the mirror one day. Intrinsic aging happens over time and regardless of resistance. Clients seen for problems such as deep smile lines or, more typically, vertical upper lip lines will report that either their mother or father has the same aging phenomenon. (See Figure 2–13.) Intrinsic aging can be influenced by disease processes as well, including autoimmune diseases such as *diabetes* or *lupus*.

While most of intrinsic aging is out of our control, it does not mean that we should throw up our hands and consider it a lost cause. Advanced skin care techniques, among them microdermabrasion in the clinical setting and sophisticated home-care regimes, can blunt the onset of the inevitable.

Extrinsic Aging

Exposure to such environmental hazards as wind, severe temperature changes, sun, smoking, and pollution accelerate the aging process and increase the potential for skin cancers.

To the clinician, extrinsic aging may be considered the type of aging that we have complete control over. We can protect our skin from extrinsic aging by using sun block or staying out of the sun altogether. Simply being outside, unprotected, will age the skin faster. Wind and extremes in temperature will age the skin faster than skin that is not exposed to temperature or wind extremes. An age-controlled comparison of an Iowa farmer's skin to that of a nongardening suburban mother who shuns the outdoors would reveal a dramatic difference in extrinsic aging.

While some body treatments are very effective in treating solar damage specifically and extrinsic aging in general, the most important task for the clinician is education of the client. All clients should be reminded of potential injuries to the skin that occur with extreme or prolonged exposure to the sun, wind, temperature extremes, and pollution. The most significant factor in extrinsic aging is exposure to the sun. (See Figure 2–14.)

Extrinsic aging magnifies **rhytids** (wrinkles), a dull, dry, and sallow appearance of the skin, actinic keratosis (overgrowth of skin layers), and irregular pigmentation. Over time, skin that is consistently exposed or has extreme exposure to the environment may develop skin cancers. While basal cell carcinomas are the most common, more serious squamous cell and **melanoma** cancers are on the rise. Recent statistics tell the story of decades of sun worship. The American Cancer Society tells us that as of this writing over one million cases of skin cancer have been diagnosed yearly. Most of these cases are considered sun related. Of the one million diagnosed cases each year, over 55,000 of those will be melanoma. Of those diagnosed with melanoma, nearly 10,000 will die.

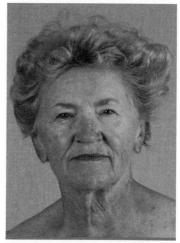

Figure 2–13 Intrinsic aging is a function of genetics

A simple yet effective way to manage extrinsic aging is to avoid smoking. It is also thought that secondhand smoke contributes to extrinsic aging.

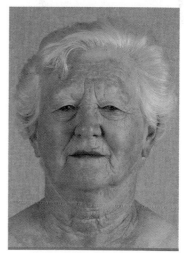

Figure 2–14 Extrinsic aging is a function of external factors such as sun exposure

rhytids
wrinkles of aging

melanoma
a malignant, darkly pigmented mole or tumor of the skin

Over time, skin that is consistently exposed or has extreme exposure to the environment may develop skin cancers.

Conclusion

On the surface the skin looks like an uncomplicated structure, simply meant to protect our inner organs from injury. But, as you can see, the skin is extraordinarily complex. There are many cells, each working to keep the skin healthy and free from infection or disease. Without a doubt you will return to this chapter to review and continue to expand your knowledge on the skin as you build your medical aesthetics career.

▶ ▷ ▷ TOP 10 TIPS TO TAKE TO THE CLINIC

1. Skin appendages include hair follicles, sweat glands, and nails and assist in epidermal healing.
2. The skin is a dynamic organ, changing daily.
3. The skin ages in two ways: intrinsically and extrinsically.
4. The epidermis is avascular.
5. The dermis houses all of the collagen, blood vessels, and nerves.
6. The keratinocyte is arguably the most important cell in the epidermis.
7. The stratum corneum (the outermost layer of the epidermis) is the layer of the skin that is "polished" by microdermabrasion.
8. The dermis and epidermis are both stimulated by microdermabrasion.
9. The stratum corneum houses the natural moisturizing factor.
10. Natural moisturizing factor is responsible for the water content in the stratum corneum, because it is able to absorb water.

CHAPTER QUESTIONS

1. What are the three layers of the skin?
2. What are the melanocytes and where are they located?
3. What are the keratinocytes and where are they located?
4. What are the appendages of the skin?
5. Why are the appendages of the skin important?
6. What are the functions of the skin?
7. Name the five layers of the epidermis.

8. Is the stratum lucidum always a part of the epidermis?

9. Name the three special cells of the epidermis.

10. What are the layers of the dermis?

11. What are the specialized cells of the dermis?

12. What is intrinsic aging?

13. What is extrinsic aging?

14. What is the natural moisturizing factor?

15. Why is the NMF important?

16. What is TEWL?

17. Why is TEWL important?

CHAPTER REFERENCES

1. Moore, E. (Ed.). (1999). *Quotation Finder*. Glascow, Scotland: Harper Collins.
2. Gray, J., MD. (1997). *The World of Skin Care*. P & G Skin Care and Research Center. Available at http://www.pg.com
3. American Society of Plastic Surgeons. (2003, December). *2002 Quick Facts on Cosmetic and Reconstructive Surgery Trends*. Available at http://www.plasticsurgery.org
4. Spense, A. P. (2004, February 22). *Basic Human Anatomy* (3rd ed.). Available at http://www.sawyerproducts.com
5. Nemours Foundation. (2004). *Skin, Hair, and Nails*. Available at http://kidshealth.org
6. Merck & Co. (2001). *Resource Library*. Available at http://www.mercksource.com
7. Ganong, W. F. (1989). Initiation of impulses in sense organs. *Review of Medical Physiology* (14th ed.). Norwalk, CT: Appleton & Lange.
8. Merck & Co. (2001). *Resource Library*. Available at http://www.mercksource.com
9. Students of Elert, G. (Ed.). (2001). *Temperature of a Healthy Human (Skin Temperature)*. Available at http://hypertextbook.com
10. Nova. (2000, November). *Surviving Denali*. Available at http://www.pbs.org
11. Gray, J., MD. (1997). *The World of Skin Care*. P & G Skin Care and Research Center. Available at http://www.pg.com
12. Gray, J., MD. (1997). *The World of Skin Care*. P & G Skin Care and Research Center. Available at http://www.pg.com

13. Gray, J., MD. (1997). *The World of Skin Care*. P & G Skin Care and Research Center. Available at http://www.pg.com

14. Gray, J., MD. (1997). *The World of Skin Care*. P & G Skin Care and Research Center. Available at http://www.pg.com

15. Nemours Foundation. (2004). *Skin, Hair, and Nails*. Available at http://kidshealth.org

16. Nemours Foundation. (2004). *Skin, Hair, and Nails*. Available at http://kidshealth.org

17. University of Iowa Healthcare. (2004, March 15). *Fluid Replacement*. Available at http://www.uihealthcare.com

18. Elsner, P., & Maibach, H. L. (Eds.). (2000). *Cosmeceuticals: Drugs vs. Cosmetics*. New York: Marcel Dekker, Inc.

19. Gray, J., MD. (1997). *The World of Skin Care*. P & G Skin Care and Research Center. Available at http://www.pg.com

20. eMedicine.com, Inc. (2004). *Hair Growth*. Available at http://www.emedicine.com

21. Nemours Foundation. (2004). *Skin, Hair, and Nails*. Available at http://kidshealth.org

22. Gray, J., MD. (1997). *The World of Skin Care*. P & G Skin Care and Research Center. Available at http://www.pg.com

23. King, D. (2003, November 14). *Introduction to Skin Histology*. Retrieved December 3, 2003, from http://www.Siumed.edu

24. Spense, A. P. (2004, February 22). *Basic Human Anatomy* (3rd ed.). Available at http://www.sawyerproducts.com

25. King, D. (2003, November 14). *Introduction to Skin Histology*. Retrieved December 3, 2003, from http://www.Siumed.edu

26. Lowe, N., MD, PhD, & Sellar, P. (1999). *Skin Secrets: The Medical Facts Versus the Beauty Fiction*. New York: Collins & Brown.

27. Baumann, L., MD. (2002). *Cosmetic Dermatology Practices and Principles*. New York: McGraw-Hill.

28. King, D. (2003, November 14). *Introduction to Skin Histology*. Retrieved December 3, 2003, from http://www.Siumed.edu

29. Baumann, L., MD. (2002). *Cosmetic Dermatology Practices and Principles*. New York: McGraw-Hill.

30. King, D. (2003, November 14). *Introduction to Skin Histology*. Retrieved December 3, 2003, from http://www.Siumed.edu

31. King, D. (2003, November 14). *Introduction to Skin Histology*. Retrieved December 3, 2003, from http://www.Siumed.edu

32. Spense, A. P. (2004, February 22). *Basic Human Anatomy* (3rd ed.). Available at http://www.sawyerproducts.com

33. Moschella, S., Pillsbury, D., & Hurley, H. (1975). *Dermatology* (Vol. 1). Philadelphia, PA: W. B. Saunders Company.

34. King, D. (2003, November 14). *Introduction to Skin Histology.* Retrieved December 3, 2003, from http://www.Siumed.edu

35. King, D. (2003, November 14). *Introduction to Skin Histology.* Retrieved December 3, 2003, from http://www.Siumed.edu

36. King, D. (2003, November 14). *Introduction to Skin Histology.* Retrieved December 3, 2003, from http://www.Siumed.edu

37. Shea, C., MD, & Prieto, V.G., MD, PhD. (2003, October 13). *Merkel Cell Carcinoma.* Available at http://www.emedicine.com

38. Baumann, L., MD. (2002). *Cosmetic Dermatology Practices and Principles.* New York: McGraw-Hill.

39. King, D. (2003, November 14). *Introduction to Skin Histology.* Retrieved December 3, 2003, from http://www.Siumed.edu

40. Spense, A. P. (2004, February 22). *Basic Human Anatomy* (3rd ed.). Available at http://www.sawyerproducts.com

41. King, D. (2003, November 14). *Introduction to Skin Histology.* Retrieved December 3, 2003, from http://www.Siumed.edu

42. King, D. (2003, November 14). *Introduction to Skin Histology.* Retrieved December 3, 2003, from http://www.Siumed.edu

43. Nemours Foundation. (2004). *Skin, Hair, and Nails.* Available at http://kidshealth.org

44. Spense, A. P. (2004, February 22). *Basic Human Anatomy* (3rd ed.). Available at http://www.sawyerproducts.com

45. Obagi, Z., MD. (2000). *Skin Health Restoration and Rejuvenation.* New York: Springer-Verlag New York, Inc.

46. Baumann, L., MD. (2002). *Cosmetic Dermatology Practices and Principles.* New York: McGraw-Hill.

47. King, D. (2003, November 14). *Introduction to Skin Histology.* Retrieved December 3, 2003, from http://www.Siumed.edu

48. King, D. (2003, November 14). *Introduction to Skin Histology.* Retrieved December 3, 2003, from http://www.Siumed.edu

49. Spense, A. P. (2004, February 22). *Basic Human Anatomy* (3rd ed.). Available at http://www.sawyerproducts.com

50. King, D. (2003, November 14). *Introduction to Skin Histology.* Retrieved December 3, 2003, from http://www.Siumed.edu

51. King, D. (2003, November 14). *Introduction to Skin Histology.* Retrieved December 3, 2003, from http://www.Siumed.edu

52. Nemours Foundation. (2004). *Skin, Hair, and Nails.* Available at http://kidshealth.org

53. Falkenbach, A. (2000). Muscle strength and vitamin D (letter). *Arch Physical and Medical Rehabilitation 81*(241).

54. Rao, D. S. (1999). Perspective on assessment of vitamin D nutrition. *Journal of Clinical Densitometry 2*(4), 457–464.

55. Obagi, Z., MD. (2000). *Skin Health Restoration and Rejuvenation*. New York: Springer-Verlag New York, Inc.

56. Bisaccia, E., MD, & Scarborough, D., MD. (2002). *The Columbia Manual of Dermatologic Cosmetic Surgery*. New York: McGraw-Hill.

Anatomy and Physiology of the Muscles

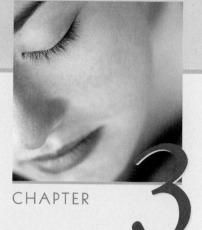

CHAPTER 3

KEY TERMS

acetylcholine
adduction
adductor group of muscles
ala
antagonist
aponeurosis
bicep brachialis
bicep brachii
cardiac fibers
cardiac muscles
deltoid
depression
elevation
endomysium
epimysium
erector spinae
extensor digitorum longus
external obliques
fibularis muscle group
flexation
frenulum
frontalis

gastrocnemius
gluteus group of muscles
hamstrings
hyperextension
insertion
intercostal muscles
internal obliques
involuntarily
lateral
latissimus dorsal
mandible
maxilla
muscle fibers
muscular system
myofilaments
nare
nasolabial
neuromuscular junction
neurons
neurotransmitter
obliquely

orifice
origin
palpebra
pectoralis major
perimysium
platysma
quadriceps
rectus abdominis
skeletal muscles
smooth muscles
soleus
sternocleidomastoids
striated
supination
synapse
tendons
tibialis anterior
trapezius
traverse abdominals
tricep brachii
voluntarily

LEARNING OBJECTIVES

After completing this chapter, you should be able to:

1. Identify the different types of muscles.
2. Explain what skeletal muscles are.
3. Identify the important muscles of the body.
4. Explain the various types of muscle movement.
5. Identify the purpose of these muscles.

51

INTRODUCTION

When we think of muscles, we tend to associate them with body builders or athletes. However, everyone has the same muscles and the same muscular structure. Our **muscular system** is a network of tissue that controls everything from digestion to walking. This specialized tissue contracts and shortens voluntarily and involuntarily to accomplish many activities. Muscle tissue is the most prevalent tissue in our bodies, accounting for half of our mass.

Many of the body treatments performed in the spa setting have a direct effect on the skeletal musculature system. Whether with a massage or hydrotherapy, a client's state of relaxation greatly depends on the condition of his or her muscles because it is in the muscular system that individuals carry their stress. In order to be accomplished at muscle manipulation and relaxation techniques associated with body treatments, the aspiring aesthetician must have a firm understanding of the skeletal muscle system.

Types of Muscles

Muscle is unique compared to other types of tissue in the body because of its ability to contract and shorten. **Myofilaments** aid this process. Muscle cells are uniquely elongated, are cylindrical in shape, and multi-nucleate. Muscle cells (except cardiac muscle cells) are referred to as **muscle fibers**.

Cumulatively, muscle cells make up three different types of specialized muscle tissue: **cardiac muscles**, **smooth muscles**, and, of most significance to the scope of this text, **skeletal muscles**. (See Figure 3–1.)

Cardiac Muscles

As the name implies, cardiac muscles are found in the heart. **Cardiac fibers** (the name for muscle cells in the heart) are unlike any other type

muscular system
complex network of tissue that supports, moves, and postures the body

myofilaments
tiny tubules that make up the muscle tissue

muscle fibers
cylindrical, multinucleated cells that can expand and contract on demand

cardiac muscles
muscle tissue type, found exclusively in the heart, and a key agent in the ability of the heart to perform

smooth muscles
type of nonstriated muscles that lines hollow cavity organs, such as the stomach and bladder, and functions to aid their operation

skeletal muscles
type of voluntary muscles that surround, protect, and move the skeletal system

cardiac fibers
flexible cells that make up cardiac muscles; found exclusively in the heart

Figure 3–1 There are three different types of muscles: skeletal muscles, cardiac muscles, and smooth muscles

of muscle tissue. They are **striated** and contract **involuntarily**, meaning we cannot consciously control their movements. The regulation of these contractions is determined by an internal pacemaker and can also be determined by the central nervous system. We will discuss the heart at greater length in Chapter 4.

Smooth Muscles

Smooth muscles are found in hollow internal organs, most often in passages where substances need a push to get through (for example, the stomach and the digestive tract). The muscle fibers have a single nucleus and lack striations. Like cardiac fibers, the muscle fibers of smooth muscles are involuntary in their movements.

Skeletal Muscles

Skeletal muscles are called this because they are attached to the skeletal system. They are the largest muscles in the body, and they are often visible to the naked eye. Located just below the skin, these muscles are a key contributor to the shape of the human form.

The muscle fibers are long and cylindrical with noticeable striations. Skeletal muscles are unique because they operate **voluntarily**. This means that a conscious decision to turn one's head will result in the head turning. Skeletal muscles can move involuntarily as well (for example, blinking). Both voluntary and involuntary movement of skeletal muscles are regulated by the brain (more on this in the following section).

Skeletal muscles can exert a great deal of force with very little effort; their inherent design allows for this. Individual muscle fibers are protected by connective tissue known as an **endomysium**. Several muscle fibers are bunched together and wrapped in a fibrous sheathing called a **perimysium**. In between these bunches, blood vessels supply nutrients and oxygen and remove waste buildup. These bunches are further supported by a tough outer sheathing known as the **epimysium**. The epimysium connects to strong connective tissue, called **tendons**, which attach the muscle to the bone.

Skeletal Muscles and the Nervous System

As already mentioned, skeletal muscles move voluntarily. When we decide to turn our heads, the result is the turning of our heads. The brain makes a conscious decision, and the muscles in our necks respond. But how is this accomplished? (See Figure 3–2.)

In simple terms, our muscles have the ability to respond to a stimulus (usually an electrical impulse sent from the brain) by contracting. Littered throughout our muscle tissue are **neurons** (nerve cells). These neurons branch out and meet muscle cells at a point called the **neuromuscular junction**. In the neuromuscular junction the nerve endings

---

striated
lined or ribbed

involuntarily
acting without thought, by way of unconscious mechanisms, or by instinct

voluntarily
acting upon free will, without instinct or coercion

endomysium
thin tissue sheath housing the muscle fibers

perimysium
connective tissue that makes up muscle fiber bundles

epimysium
outer layer of connective tissue sheathing a muscle

tendons
fibrous and tough fiber that connects muscle tissue to a bone or joint

neurons
nervous system cells that process and transmit nerve impulses

neuromuscular junction
point where muscles interpret nerve impulses into voluntary muscle movement

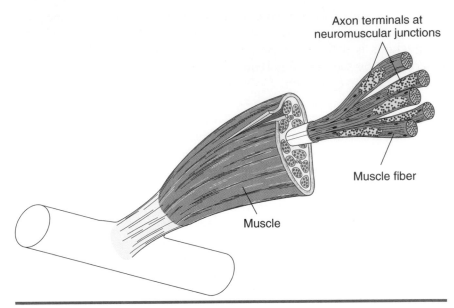

Axon terminals at neuromuscular junctions

Muscle fiber

Muscle

Figure 3–2 Skeletal muscles move voluntarily

and the muscle fibers never quite touch one another. In between is the **synapse**. A **neurotransmitter**, called **acetylcholine** (ACh), crosses the synapse and is received on the other end. Once ACh reaches its port of reception, a chemical reaction produces an electrical current that travels the length of the muscle cell. Because muscle fibers have the ability to respond to a stimulus, a property known as irritability, the response is the contraction of the muscle fiber. Cumulatively, the response is the shortening of the muscle, and hence, the desired motion intended by the original conscious decision.

Function of Skeletal Muscles

Our muscles do not just serve the singular purpose of movement. In fact, they are multifunctional. Muscles help us maintain upright posture, stabilize joints, generate heat, and hold our internal organs in place.

Movement is necessary, but what is truly splendid with regards to movement is instinctual motion. Instinctual motion saves us from hurting ourselves. Consider touching something that is hot. Before the pain truly registers, we unconsciously pull our hands away from the heat. While our conscious minds could realize the pain and remove our hands as well, this instinctive motion means the difference between a superficial burn and deep thermal injury.

Movement is something that usually comes easily and is often taken for granted. Without the ability to move, we could not eat, breathe, talk, walk, or even smile. The ability to "do" is thanks to our muscles.

We also owe our upright posture to our muscles. While gravity is constantly trying to pull us down, our muscles are actively resisting. This allows us to stand up, jump, walk, and sit down at will. Even the mere act of standing requires our muscles to perform complex tasks in conjunction with our brains. We truly notice the role our muscles play in posture when our posture is poor. Repeated exposure to poor ergonomic conditions causes our muscles to overcompensate and become strained and tense over time. As an aspiring aesthetician, injuring your body could be career threatening.

Our muscles also work very closely with our skeletal system, our joints in particular. The strength of muscles and tendons compensate for some inherent design flaws in our joints. This allows the joints to function over longer periods of time.

One of the less mentioned but vital duties of the muscles is the production of heat. We have all heard that energy is neither created nor destroyed. The same is true for the body. The energy that creates the kinetic energy of our movements is mostly converted to heat. This heat, in turn, is important to maintain our ideal body temperature.

With regard to terminology, as we advance into the specific muscles throughout the body, it is important to explain some of the terms used. All muscles have a beginning point, which is called the **origin**. Similarly, all muscles have an end point, which is called the **insertion**. These terms will be used throughout this chapter. Also, muscles control movements, and each of these movements has a name. See Table 3–1 for a detailed list of these movements.

origin
point where a given muscle begins

insertion
muscle end point

■ MUSCLES OF THE HEAD AND FACE

Our faces are wrought with expression, as we know. These expressions have their origins in the muscles that lie beneath the skin.

Muscles of the Forehead

The skin of the scalp is among the thickest types of skin of the body. Hair follicles cover much of it, particularly over the scalp, and over its entirety are found a few (during adolescence we may think way too many) sebaceous glands.

The scalp adheres closely to fascia and underlying muscle, and movements of those muscles move our skin. We have no muscles underneath the scalp proper. Muscles of the forehead and temple fan out into fascia in the direction of the crown.

Table 3–1	Types of Body Movement
Flexation	To move the joint in such a way as to decrease the angle of the joint
Extension	To move the joint in such a way as to increase the angle of the joint
Hyperextension	If the extension is greater than 180 degrees it is considered hyperextension
Rotation	A movement of ball and socket joints
Abduction	Moving the limb away from the center of the body
Adduction	Moving the limb to the center of the body
Circumduction	A combination of many movements including flexion, extension, abduction, adduction
Dorsiflexion	Moving up or down as in the foot
Inversion	Related to the foot; turning the sole to the center of the body
Eversion	The opposite of inversion
Supination	To turn backward
Pronation	To turn forward
Opposition	As the thumb touches the fingers

frontalis
muscle that makes up the forehead

aponeurosis
the tendon-like structure that actually connects the tendon to the bone

The forehead musculature is simple. There is only one muscle, the **frontalis**. While the frontalis is a single muscle, it can behave as if it were two muscles or at least bifurcated; but it is not. You no doubt have seen expressions where only half of the forehead was used, a lift of one eyebrow, for example. The frontalis (see Figure 3–3) lies directly beneath the skin of our forehead, stretching from temple to temple and from the eyebrow to approximately the hairline. (See Figure 3–4.) At the hairline, the frontalis shades off into an **aponeurosis** with the thick fascia of the vertex of the skull.

As you might expect, the frontalis is responsible for lifting the eyebrows. At the same time, it works to draw the scalp forward, producing transverse or horizontal wrinkles.

Although as a muscle it stands practically alone, the frontalis is still a team player. In its lower middle it blends into the procerus, a muscle of the nose; to each side it blends with the upper eye muscles, the corrugator and orbicularis oculi. The nerve powering the frontalis muscle is a branch of the facial nerve aptly called the frontal branch.

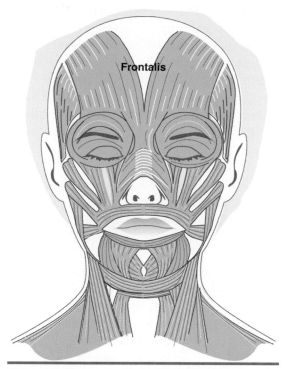

Figure 3–3 The frontalis lies directly beneath the skin of our forehead and is responsible for the expressions of the forehead

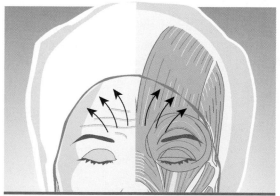

Figure 3–4 The frontalis is responsible for lifting the eyebrows

Muscles of the Eyes

We come now to the periocular area, the muscles of the area around our eyes. Two muscles lying beneath our eyebrows and over our eyes help control our expressions. As time passes, our habitual expressions tend to become rather well tracked into our faces.

Our eyelids and eyebrows are mobile because of these muscles: the orbicularis oculi, the levator palpebrae superioris, and the corrugator supercilii. If you know any Latin, you will recognize that the orbicularis has to do with orb, so it must involve the eye; the levator has to do with lifting. *Super-* means above and the Latin word *cilium* means eyelash; "supercilia" is plural and means above the eyelashes. As for corrugator —think cardboard. (See Figure 3–5.)

Let us take these muscles in order. The orbicularis oculi starts from the nose and wraps over the orb of the eye to form the eyelid, or **palpebra**, and finally fans out toward the temple. It is a sphincter muscle, meaning that it contracts to close an **orifice**, the eye. The muscle acts involuntarily to close the eye, as in sleeping or blinking, and we also move it voluntarily. When the entire muscle is worked, as when you shut your eyes tightly, the skin of the forehead, temple, and cheek is pulled together, causing folds to radiate from the outside or **lateral** angle of the eyelid. As we age, these folds become permanent and are called crow's feet. (See Figure 3–6.)

The levator palpebrae superioris antagonizes, or works against, the orbicularis oculi, as it raises the upper eyelid to expose the orb of the eye. And the corrugator? This aptly named muscle is the "frowning" muscle, drawing the eyebrow down and toward the middle and producing those vertical wrinkles we know so well. (See Figure 3–7.)

Muscles of the Mouth

Many muscles are involved in the movement of the mouth and cheek area. We will concentrate on those that produce our characteristic expressions and their consequent lines. (See Table 3–2.)

palpebra
the eyelid

orifice
a hole or opening

lateral
located on the side

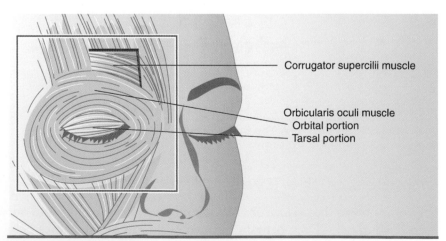

Figure 3–5 Orbicularis oculi encircles the eye

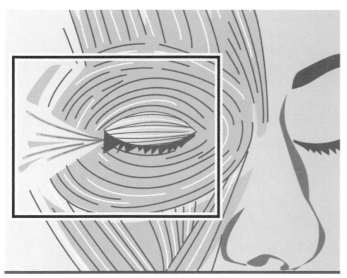

Figure 3–6 The movement of the orbicularis oculi causes crow's feet to develop

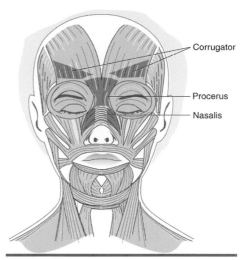

Figure 3–7 The glabellar muscles include corrugator, procerus, and pyramidalis nasi

The quadratus labii superioris is a broad sheet of muscle extending from the side of the nose and the upper lip to the zygomatic, or cheek, bone. This muscle elevates the upper lip, at the same time pushing it a little bit forward. Parts of this muscle help to form the **nasolabial** furrow, sometimes known not so fondly as "marionette lines," the lines passing from the side of the nose to the upper lip, imparting an expression of sadness. When the whole muscle works, pushing the lip out farther, it causes an expression of contempt or disdain.

Levator labii superioris and levator anguli oris—these muscles of the upper lip raise the angle of the mouth. Their combined efforts assist in forming the nasolabial ridge, that pesky line passing from the side of the

nasolabial
pertaining to the nose and mouth

Table 3–2	Major Muscles of the Mouth	
Above the Mouth	**Below the Mouth**	**Around the Mouth**
Quadratus labii superioris	Levator labii Inferioris	Orbicularis oris
Levator labii superioris	Depressor anguli oris	Mentalis
Levator anguli oris	Depressor labii inferior	Quadratus labii Inferioris
Zygomaticus		Risorius
		Buccinator

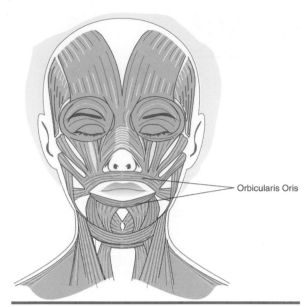

Orbicularis Oris

Figure 3–8 The mouth has many muscles that cause a variety of movements

nose to the upper lip. This line can be an indication of age based on its depth and surrounding tissue laxity. (See Figure 3–8.)

The zygomaticus attaches to the front of the zygomatic bone—hence its name—and descends **obliquely** until it inserts into the angle of the mouth. It draws the angle of the mouth back and upward when we laugh.

The levator labii inferioris, controls the lower lip, raising the lower lip and making it protrude. That causes the skin of the chin to wrinkle in a pout.

With the depressor anguli oris and depressor labii inferioris, think "to depress." These muscles of the lower jaw and lower lip give further expression to movements of the lower lip. The depressor labii inferioris draws the lower lip down and a little out, giving an expression of irony. The depressor anguli oris is the **antagonist** to the levator anguli oris; instead of pushing the lower lip forward, it draws it down and back, as if you had just tasted something bitter.

The orbicularis oris encircles the mouth, but is not a simple sphincter muscle. It consists of many layers or strata of muscular tissue surrounding the orifice of the mouth but having opposing actions. It also attaches and blends into neighboring facial muscles. Its most common action is to close the lips; its deep fibers compress the lips against the alveolar arch of the teeth, as when someone is trying to feed you something that you do not want. The superficial part of the orbicularis oris can also protrude the closed lips forward.

obliquely
situated at a slant

antagonist
a muscle or muscle group that counteracts the motions of the agonist counterpart

The mentalis is a small bundle of muscle fibers at the side of the **frenulum** of the lower lip. A frenulum is a tissue that connects one thing to another—a frenulum, for example, attaches the bottom of the tongue to the floor of the mouth. The frenulum of the lower lip attaches it to the gums. The mentalis muscle raises and protrudes the lower lip as it wrinkles the skin of the chin, producing an expression of doubt or disdain. The quadratus labii inferioris, arising from the **mandible** to insert into the lower lip, draws that lip down and somewhat to the side, producing an expression of irony.

The risorius begins over the masseter, the muscle used in chewing, and passes horizontally forward to insert into the angle of the mouth. It retracts downward the angle of the mouth, producing an unpleasant grinning expression.

The name "buccinators" comes from the Latin *buccina,* meaning a trumpet. It is formed at the outer surfaces of the **maxilla** and mandible at about the level of the three molar teeth. Its fibers converge into the angle of the mouth, and its action is to compress the cheeks so that, as we chew, the food is kept at the mercy of our teeth. After we distend our cheeks with air, the buccinator muscles can expel it from between the lips in a whistle or a trumpet blow. All of these facial muscles are supplied by the facial nerve, cranial nerve VII. (See Figure 3–9.)

Nasal Muscles

While on the subject of frowning, we will introduce the procerus, a muscle of the nose, which draws up the nose and pushes down the central

frenulum
a small tissue that anchors a mucous membrane to surrounding tissue

mandible
the lower portion of the jaw

maxilla
the upper portion of the jaw

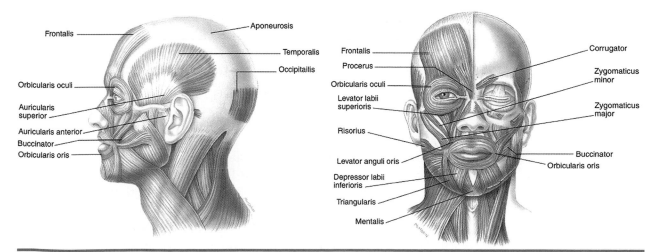

Figure 3–9 The major muscles of the head and face

brow area. Just below is the pyramidalis nasi, which, as you might imagine, is shaped like a pyramid over the nasal bone. It draws down the inner angle of the eyelids to make transverse "squinting" wrinkles across the nose. Just below that, on the side of the nose and extending between the inner margin of the eye and the upper lip, lies a small triangular muscle with a truly impressive name, the levator labii superioris alaeque nasi. The purpose of this little muscle is to push upward the upper lip and **ala**, the flaring expansion on the side of each **nare**, or nostril. This causes a noticeable dilation of the nose and a wrinkling upon its ridge, the effect of which is a marked expression of contempt or disdain.

■ MUSCLES OF THE NECK

The muscles of the neck have a heavy load to carry: They support the head and all the valuable contents contained within. They provide rotational movement of the head, an act without which our safety would be compromised on many levels. There are, in fact, many muscles that work the neck; however, only two, the sternocleidomastoid and the platysma, are relevant to the scope of this text.

Sternocleidomastoid

The **sternocleidomastoids** are found on either side of the neck. They act to flex and rotate the head. Sometimes referred to as "prayer muscles," they are charged with lowering the head when they act together, or rotating the head in either direction.

The sternocleidomastoids are considered "dual headed" muscles, meaning they are broad at their points of origin (the sternum on one side and the clavicle on the other) and destination (the temporal bone), and tapered in the middle. These muscles contain a lot of stress and are often the source of stress headaches due to their proximity to major blood vessels that supply blood to the brain.

Platysma

The **platysma** is a superficial muscle that originates in the chest area and ends just below the chin. Its sheath-like form is responsible for the external contours of the neck. This muscle crisscrosses both the trapezius and the sternocleidomastoid. The main duties of this muscle are pulling the corners of the mouth downward and supporting and balancing the upright head. (See Figure 3–10.)

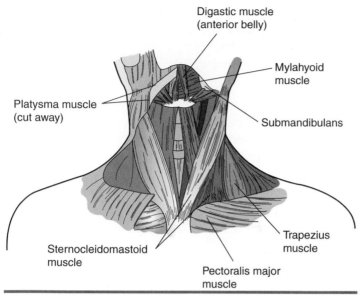

Figure 3–10 There are many muscles of the neck and chest, but the sternocleidomastoid and the platysma are the most important muscles for the aesthetician to know

■ MUSCLES OF THE TRUNK

The trunk of the body, or the thorax, is where all the meat is contained. It houses the vital organs of our bodies and provides many more essential functions, including balance. Within the trunk there are several muscle groups that provide balance and upright posture and fight gravity. These muscles are subcategorized into their position on the body, anterior or posterior.

Anterior Muscles of the Trunk

Anterior muscles are those that are on the front of the body. They provide balance, contribute to the operation of the limbs, and provide support for vital organ systems contained within.

Pectoral Muscles

The muscles of the upper chest consist mostly of the **pectoralis major**. This large convergent muscle resembles a fan. Its point of origin is broad. It begins at the sternum, clavicle, and ribs. The destination point is much narrower and inserts into the crest of the greater tubercle of the humerus

pectoralis major
prominent muscles of the upper chest

flexation
the ability of a muscle or muscle group to bend a limb at a central joint

adduction
the ability to move inward

intercostal muscles
short muscles that fill in the gaps between the ribs, aiding respiration

traverse abdominals
innermost layer of abdominal muscles

internal obliques
inner layer of muscles that line the abdomen

external obliques
outermost layer of muscle tissue lining the abdomen

rectus abdominis
horizontally paired muscles running down the length of the abdomen

(the bone that runs shoulder to elbow). These muscles are primarily responsible for the upward (**flexation**) and side-to-side (**adduction**) movement of the upper limbs.

Intercostal Muscles

Intercostal muscles are found between the ribs, and there are two kinds: the *internal* and *external* intercostals. The internal intercostal muscles (in the inside of the rib case) extend from the front of the ribs and go around back, past the bend in the ribs. The external intercostal muscles (on the outside of the rib case) wrap around from the back of the rib almost to the end of the bony part of the rib in front. The intercostal muscles are comparatively small and play a vital role in providing movement of the rib cage to allow breathing.

Abdominal Muscles

The abdominal muscles sit on the front and sides of the lower half of the torso, originating along the rib cage and attaching along the pelvis. The abdominal region houses major organ systems that the muscles hold in place. These systems include the urinary system and the digestive system, as well as the internal components of the reproductive system.

The muscles that form the abdominal group include traverse abdominals, the internal and external obliques, and the rectus abdominis. These muscles serve a variety of tasks ranging from forced breathing to excretion. They lay one on top of each other and run in differing directions, allowing for the most support for the internal organs within.

The **traverse abdominals** are the deepest of the abdominal muscles. Their side-to-side striations compress the internal organs. They originate at the lower ribs and end at the pelvis.

The next abdominal layer is the **internal obliques**. They run at obtuse angles to the traverse abdominal muscles. Along with the **external obliques** above, the major functions of these muscles are movement of the vertebrae and rotation of the trunk.

The outermost layer is the **rectus abdominis**. These are paired side by side, with vertical striations. These are the muscles that compose the sought-after "six pack." They are responsible for vertebrae movement, forced breathing, as well as the specialized tasks of childbirth.

Posterior Muscles of the Trunk

Posterior muscles are those that are located on the back of the body. They provide balance, contribute to the operation of the limbs, and provide support for vital organ systems contained within.

Trapezius

The **trapezius** is a diamond shaped coupling of superficial muscles that make up the majority of our upper backs. They originate at the occipital bone of the skull and run down through the thoracic vertebrae. Their insertion point is on the scapula. They are responsible for a wide range of motion of the back and shoulders. This includes scapular **elevation** (shrugging up), scapular adduction (drawing the shoulder blades together), and scapular **depression** (pulling the shoulder blades down).

Latissimus Dorsal

If the trapezius comprises the majority of muscle tissue on the upper back, the **latissimus dorsal** comprises most of the muscle tissue on the lower back. Like the pectoralis major on the anterior side, the latissimus dorsal is fan shaped with a broad origin and a relatively small insertion point. The latissimus dorsal originates along the lower spine and finds its destination along the posterior side of the humerus. These muscles are especially useful for rotational movement of the arms.

Erector Spinae

Those who suffer from back pain are acutely aware of the **erector spinae** muscle group. This set of three muscles runs along either side of the spinal column. Their chief responsibility is to protect upright positioning and to act as the antagonist muscle in the action of bending from the waist.

■ MUSCLES OF THE ARMS AND SHOULDERS

The muscles of the arms and shoulders are both powerful and resourceful. After all, without these muscles, we would not be able to do most of the things that separate us from other animals. Anatomically speaking, the arm is the region of the body from the shoulder joint to the elbow joint. The forearm is the section from the elbow to the wrist. However, collectively, they are commonly referred to as the arm. The major muscles found in the collective arm are the **deltoid**, the **bicep brachii**, the **bicep brachialis**, and the **tricep brachii**.

The Deltoid

The deltoid is a triangle shaped muscle that forms the rounded contour of the shoulder. It is an extremely fleshy muscle and serves to protect and aid

trapezius
two flat fleshy muscles that span either side of the upper back, allowing for movement of the head and shoulders

elevation
ability to rise vertically

depression
an area of skin that is lower than surrounding tissue

latissimus dorsal
large flat muscles that span the back

erector spinae
long muscle that spans the length of the back and neck; key component to upright posturing

deltoid
triangular muscle found in the shoulder that raises the arms to the side

bicep brachii
the muscle of the arm that bends the upper arm and turns the hand over

bicep brachialis
fleshy muscle of the upper arm that is responsible for flexing the elbow and rotating the arm

tricep brachii
large muscle that runs along the underside of the upper arm and extends the arm

hyperextension
extension of a bodily joint beyond the
normal range of motion

supination
to rotate a joint a complete 180°; for
example, rotating the wrist such that
the hand faces forward then backward

the shoulder joint, as well as to provide arm abduction and shoulder **hyperextension**. It originates at the clavicle and is inserted at the humerus. Because of the fleshy nature of this muscle, it is a preferred location to inject intramuscular medications.

The Bicep Brachii

As far as muscles go, none are more recognizable than the bicep brachii, or just bicep. In fact, it has become a symbol for fitness and musculature. The name "bicep" literally means "two heads," because it originates from two heads attached to the scapula (collarbone) and the humerus. The main duties of this muscle are flexation and **supination** (rotation of the arm). When it contracts, it works to flex the forearm at the elbow.

Because of the iconic nature of the muscle, those who lift weights work this muscle hard. It is also a muscle that responds well to such workouts. In fact, it can grow up to 30 inches in height.

The Brachialis

Below the bicep is the brachialis. Although the bicep gets all the attention, the brachialis is equally important for the arm's ability to flex at the elbow. Its origin is at the deltoid muscle and it inserts at the lower half of the humerus. (See Figure 3–11 and Table 3–3.)

Triceps Brachii

Just as the biceps have two heads, the triceps have three heads, as the name implies. It originates from the shoulder and the humerus, inserting in the ulna. It is a superficial muscle that is tasked with extension of the arm and elbow. This muscle allows us to hold our arms out in front of us.

MUSCLES OF THE LEGS

Our legs are tasked with moving and carrying our entire bodies. Our legs are where we find some of largest, densest muscle tissue in our bodies. This is in part because they carry a huge load. These muscles move our legs in coordination with three joints: the hip, the knees, and the ankle. (See Figure 3–12.)

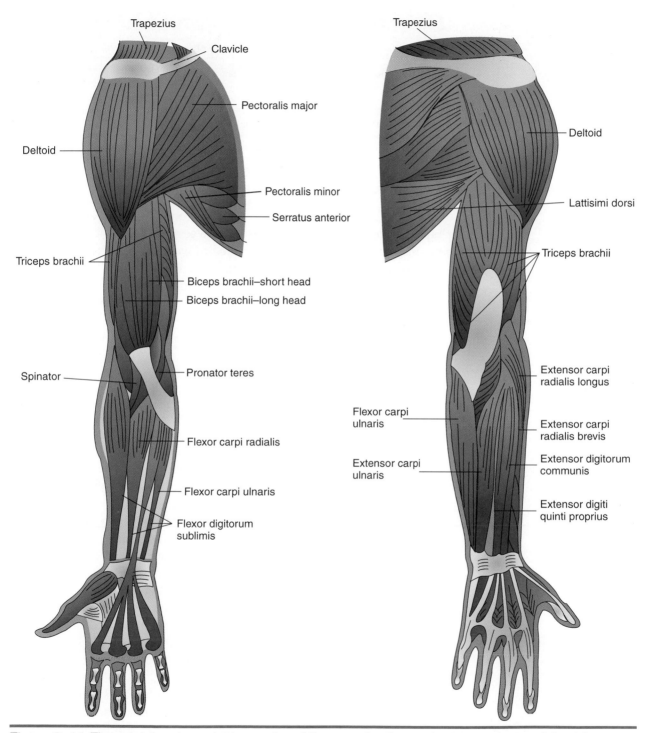

Figure 3–11 There are four important muscles of the arms for the aesthetician to know: deltoid, bicep brachii, bicep brachialis, and tricep brachii

Table 3–3	Muscles of the Arms and Their Movement
Deltoid	arm abduction and shoulder hyperextension
Bicep Brachii	flexation and supination of the arm
Bicep Brachialis	flexes the elbow
Tricep Brachii	extension of the arm and elbow

Leg Muscles Associated with the Hip

The hip is a remarkable joint. It holds our bodies upright and allows for biped posture. While it is not as flexible as other joints, its sturdiness is necessary and impressive. The limited movement is powerful, nonetheless. Walking, standing upright, and balancing on one leg are accomplished because of subtle contractions of muscles that regulate the hip. There are five muscle groups that regulate hip movement: rotators, adductors, abductors, flexors, and extensors. Because of the limited scope of this text, we will place our emphasis on the larger more superficial muscles.

Gluteus Group of Muscles

Probably the most well known of the muscle groups in the lower limbs, the **gluteus group of muscles** together forms the exterior contours of our buttocks. Aside from the important movements they allow for, they also provide cushioning that protects our hips and spine when we sit or lay down. These fleshy muscles are named according to their size, and all have varying duties.

The largest one, the gluteus maximus, has its origin at the hip and connects to the femur. Its major task is to maintain a safe alignment with the femur. This is important for activities such as climbing. The gluteus maximus is considered part of the hip extensors.

Next is the gluteus medius. It is located below the gluteus maximus, connecting at the ilium and inserting in the femur on either side of the leg. It is considered to be both a rotator and an abductor. It functions to provide support for this hip while walking or running and also during hip rotation. Due in part to their frequent use, these muscles are often subject to stress buildup.

Finally, the brevis is a coupling of muscles that work in conjunction with the gluteus medius, primarily for hip rotation. A small muscle (as the name implies), its origin is found in the ilium, and its insertion is in the upper femur.

gluteus group of muscles
muscle group that makes up the uppermost thigh and lowermost trunk

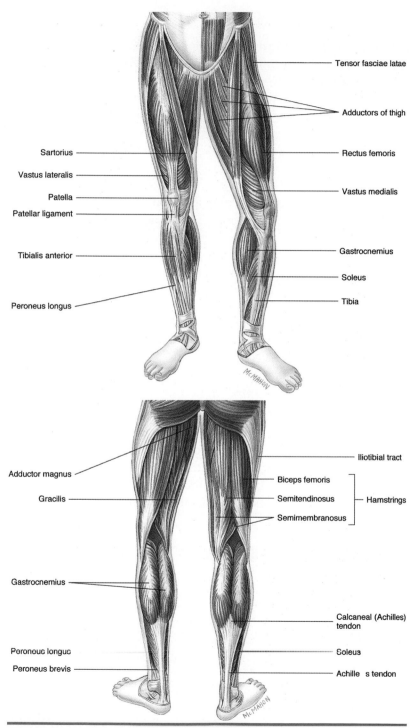

Figure 3–12 The muscles of the legs are large, to accommodate the weight of the body

Adductor Group of Muscles

The **adductor group of muscles** includes smaller muscles that work to keep the legs together during most physical activity. The adductor magnus, longus, brevis, and pectineus make up the adductor group. Their origin is at the hip or pelvic bone, and the insertion point is at the knee joint. Groin pulls are a strain at the attachment of the adductors to the pubic bone. (See Table 3–4.)

Muscles Associated with the Knee

The main movements of the knee are flexion and extension. Several groups of muscles make this possible. Obviously the knee is one of the most used joints and is subject to much strain over time. Also in the knee, there are some vital ligaments that affect movement. Athletes are particularly subject to tears in these ligaments, which can be extremely painful. While the ligaments are crucial to the flexation and extension performed by the knee, the muscles do all the heavy lifting. While there are many muscles that participate in knee movement, the scope of this text justifies the discussion of only a few superficial muscles and muscle groups.

The Posterior Thigh (Hamstrings)

On the top or posterior side of the thigh is a muscle group called the **hamstrings**. These three muscles, the biceps femoris, the semitendinosus, and the semimembranosus, control the pull on the knee joint, or flexation of the knee. They originate at the ischial tuberosity, on the lower pelvis, and insert at the tibia. This muscle group consists of large and strong muscles that are responsible for the external contours of the front of the thigh.

Table 3–4 Muscles of the Legs and Their Function	
Gluteus maximus	hip extensor
Gluteus medius	hip rotator
Gluteus minimus	hip rotator
Adductor magnus	leg abduction
Adductor longus	leg abduction
Adductor brevis	leg abduction
Adductor pectineus	leg abduction

The Anterior Thigh (Quadraceps)

Whereas the hamstrings regulate flexation of the knee, the **quadriceps**, located on the anterior, or rear, of the thigh regulate extension. As the name might imply, there are four muscles in this muscle group: the rectus femoris, the vastus medalis, the vastus lateralis, and the vastus intermedius. The most superficial of these muscles is the rectus feoris, which originates at the pelvis. The vastus muscles, which lay below and to either side, originate from the femur. All four muscles in this group insert in the knee by way of the patellar ligament. The rectus femoris acts as a flexor muscle for the hip, and all four act to extend the knee. This is a very powerful group of muscles, even on persons who are less athletic.

Muscles Associated with the Ankle and Foot

No place in our bodies has as many bones as the foot and ankle. This network of many tiny bones works in conjunction with several ligaments and small muscles that perform a variety of motions for the foot. Since the feet act as our contact with the ground on which we walk, a lot of emphasis is placed on shock absorption in this region. (See Figure 3–13 and Table 3–5.)

The Tibialis Anterior

Situated on the length of the inside of the tibia bone, the **tibialis anterior** is a vital muscle for controlling dorsiflexion of the foot. It originates just below the knee and inserts at the base of the first metatarsal bone of the foot. At its point of origination, the tibialis anterior muscle is fleshy but thins out toward its end, becoming tendonous.

The Extensor Digitorum Longus

The **extensor digitorum longus** is a thin long muscle that runs the length of the side of the tibialis anterior muscle. Between the two muscles exist a few vital nerves. It originates just below the knee and inserts between the third and fourth toes. It is responsible for lifting the second through fifth toes as well as for dorsiflexion of the ankle.

The Fibularis Muscle Group

The **fibularis muscle group**, also called the peronaeus muscle group, consists of three muscles, the tertius peronaeus, peronaeus longus, and the peronaeus brevis. The first one, the tertius peronaeus, is a small muscle that is considered to be part of the extensor digitorium longus.

quadriceps
large muscle at the top of the thigh responsible for extending the leg

tibialis anterior
long muscle that runs the length of the tibia and maneuvers the foot

extensor digitorum longus
thin, long muscle of the lower leg; responsible for extending the four smallest toes, and pronates the foot

fibularis muscle group
group of muscles that spans the length of the fibula in the lower legs

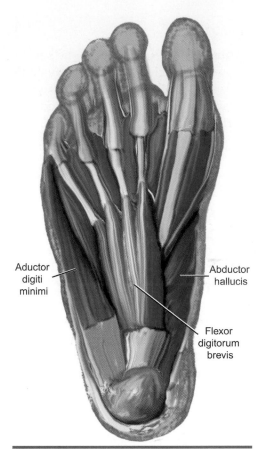

Aducter
digiti
minimi

Abductor
hallucis

Flexor
digitorum
brevis

Figure 3–13 The muscles of the feet play an important role in support of the ankle and the leg

Interestingly, not all individuals have this muscle. It begins below the outside of the knee and inserts into the little toe. The second one, the peronaeus longus, is a superficial muscle that runs along the side of the fibula. The third muscle of this group, the peronaeus brevis, lies below the peronaeus longus. It originates around the same place as the peronaeus longus, just below the knee, and inserts at the ankle. Collectively, this group of muscles moves the ankle.

The Gastrocnemius

Most people are familiar with the **gastrocnemius**, even though they may not know it. That is because most people know it as the "calf muscle." It

gastrocnemius
commonly called the "calf" muscle; responsible for extending the foot and flexing the knee

Table 3–5   Muscles of the Feet and Their Functions

Tibialis anterior	dorsiflexion of the foot
Extensor digitorum longus	dorsiflexion of the ankle
Tertius peronaeus	dorsiflexion of the ankle
Peronaeus longus	dorsiflexion of the ankle
Peronaeus brevis	dorsiflexion of the ankle
Gastrocnemius	plantar flex the foot; flexation of the knee
Soleus	plantar flex the foot

originates from two heads, just above the rear of the knee, and inserts along with the soleus into the calcaneus tendon, or "Achilles heel." These powerful muscles are critical to the function of walking. The calf muscle acts to plantar flex the foot, and also plays a secondary role in flexation of the knee. Since there exist several major blood vessels housed within the calf, it plays a major role in peripheral venous return (see Chapter 4) when in the upright position.

The Soleus

Some professionals consider the **soleus** to be part of the calf. However, this powerful muscle is vital to the functions of standing and walking, so, therefore, it deserves its due credit. Located on the back of the leg, this fleshy superficial muscle originates at the fibula and inserts at the calcaneus tendon at the heel. Like the gastrocneminus, the soleus acts to plantar flex the foot. Different from the gastrocneminus, the soleus plays an important role in posture, supporting the ankle, and the leg as a whole.

soleus
long muscle situated under the "calf" muscles

Conclusion

Because body treatments performed in a spa will have a noticeable result on muscles, it is important to know the muscles that will be affected. Because of the daily rigors of normal life, our muscle tissue is often subject to stress buildup. The exact muscles that will receive the stress buildup will vary from person to person, which is why it is valuable to the aspiring aesthetician to have a fundamental knowledge of the major muscles found in the human bodies.

▶ ⟩ ⟩ ⟩ TOP 10 TIPS TO TAKE TO THE CLINIC

1. There are three types of muscles: cardiac muscles, smooth muscles, and skeletal muscles.
2. Skeletal muscles are called this because they are attached to the skeletal system.
3. Skeletal muscles move voluntarily.
4. Muscles help us maintain upright posture, stabilize joints, generate heat, and hold our internal organs in place.
5. All muscles have a beginning point that is called the origin. Similarly, all muscles have an end point that is called the insertion.
6. The trunk of the body, or the thorax, is where all the meat is contained.
7. Our legs are where we find some of largest, densest muscle tissue in our bodies.
8. The muscles of the arm and shoulder are both powerful and resourceful.
9. The main movements of the knee are flexion and extension. Several groups of muscles make this possible.
10. Since the feet act as our contact with the ground on which we walk, a lot of emphasis is placed on shock absorption.

CHAPTER QUESTIONS

1. What are muscle fibers?
2. What types of muscle tissue are found in humans?
3. Do cardiac muscles move voluntarily or involuntarily? What about skeletal muscles?
4. What functions do skeletal muscles serve?
5. What is the point where muscles begin? End? What purposes do neck muscles serve?
6. What is adduction? Flexation?
7. What purposes do trunk muscles serve?
8. What do trapezius muscles do?
9. What major muscles are found in the arm? What do they do?
10. Which muscles assist in the hip movement/support?
11. Where are adductor muscles?
12. What roles do soleus muscles serve?

Anatomy and Physiology of the Cardiovascular System

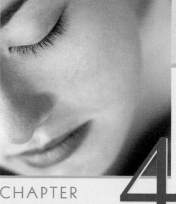

 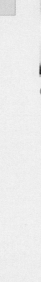

KEY TERMS

agranulocytes
albumin
anastomosis
anemia
antibodies
aorta
aortic semilunar valve
arteries
arterioles
atria
atrioventricular valves
basophils
bicuspid valve
blood pressure
capillaries
cardiovascular system
clotting factors
collateral circulation
cylindrical
deoxygenated
desiccation
diastole

edema
electrolytes
eosinophils
epicardium
erythrocytes
flexor
formed elements
granulocytes
heart disease
hemoglobin
hemophilia
hydrostatic pressure
hypoxia
leukemia
leukocytes
ligature
lymph
lymph nodes
lymphatic drainage
lymphatic vessels
lymphocytes
monocytes

myocardium
neutrophils
oxygenated
pericardium
peripheral edema
phagocytes
plasma
platelets
plexuses
pulmonary circulation
pulmonary valve
semilunar valves
stethoscope
systemic circulation
systole
thalassemia
tortuous
tricuspid valve
varicose veins
veins
ventricles

LEARNING OBJECTIVES

After completing this chapter, you should be able to:

1. Identify the difference between veins and arteries.
2. Describe and list all of the parts of the cardiovascular system.
3. Name three important facts about the blood.
4. Name five cells found in the blood.

75

INTRODUCTION

While it is important that all of the body's systems work in harmony, each is important in its own way. In this chapter we will explore the circulatory system and, in particular, the veins and arteries.

The **veins** and **arteries** are most commonly thought of for the transportation of blood from the heart to the tissues and organs and back to the heart again. But as with each system in the body, the circulatory system is at risk for disease and injury. When we think of diseases of the circulatory system, we normally think of heart disease or heart attacks. In this chapter we focus on the veins and arteries and one particular condition that affects nearly 50 percent of the population, varicose veins. In fact, half of the women reading this textbook will have some variation of varicose veins: spider veins in some form or large scale varicosities. But before we begin our discussion about varicose veins, we need to understand the normal anatomy and physiology of veins and arteries and how they relate to the circulatory system at large.

■ THE CARDIOVASCULAR SYSTEM

At the center of the **cardiovascular system** or circulatory system, sits the heart, a hollow muscle that really does not sit at all. Throughout our lives it constantly pumps blood, through contraction and relaxation movements, to all parts of the body through a sinuous series of tubes called arteries. Arteries branch out into smaller and smaller vessels, finally ending in **arterioles**, which in turn open into a sieve of microscopic vessels called capillaries. After the blood passes through the capillaries, it begins its homeward route by entering venules, the smallest branches of veins, the vessels that return blood to the heart. Generally speaking, one can say that the arteries contain oxygen and nutrients while veins carry deoxygenated blood and metabolic waste.

The veins and arteries start out flexible and pliant, but as we age they may become less flexible. We cannot help the slow march of time, but some things we do have control over. We all understand the importance of keeping cholesterol levels and blood pressure in check, and if we do not know which foods are heart healthy, the information is readily available for anyone seeking it. You may know that smoking is bad for the lungs, but did you know that smoking limits the capacity of the circulatory system, contributing to inflexibility in the vessels and **desiccation** of the capillaries? This not only impairs blood and oxygen exchange but slows healing, and may make postsurgical scarring more prominent.

---

veins
carry unoxygenated blood to the lungs

arteries
network of tubes that transport oxygenated blood to tissues, organs, and cells

cardiovascular system
the entirety of the heart and blood vessel system

arterioles
smallest component of the arteries that connects with capillary beds

desiccation
removal of all fluids

The fluid that is pumped by the heart through the veins and arteries is blood. Therefore, it is the logical place to begin our tour of the circulatory system.

■ BLOOD

While the thought of, and the sight of, blood is repellant to some, it is an unmistakable necessity to every cell, tissue, organ, and system of the human body. Blood is of such fantastic and life sustaining value that it has become a cultural symbol representing life and death, pain and healing, horror and beauty, and everything in between. Almost every form of spirituality possesses its own representations of blood and its value.

From a scientific perspective, blood is equally significant. It transports the requisite components to where they are needed, while redistributing the useless and harmful components to where they can be properly disposed. In addition to nutrient supply, gas exchange, and waste disposal, the blood is actively engaged in almost every function of the body. Thermoregulation, wound healing, and immunologic responses are just a few. With so much to accomplish, it is easy to see why blood is considered the fluid of life. (See Table 4–1.)

Blood Composition

As mentioned above, blood is considered a fluid tissue. While it appears to the naked eye as a liquid, it also has solid and gaseous properties. This versatility allows blood to accomplish its varied tasks as needed. The liquid component, **plasma**, is a yellowish fluid that accounts for just a little more than half of the blood's volume. Plasma is 90 to 95 percent water, and the remaining 5 to 10 percent consists of proteins and trace minerals, including **albumin**, **clotting factors**, **antibodies**, and **electrolytes**. (See Table 4–2.)

The second component of blood is the **formed elements**. (See Table 4–3.) Formed elements are specialized blood cells that are suspended in the liquid (plasma) vehicle. In total, formed elements make up just under half of blood's total volume. The vast majority of these are **erythrocytes**, commonly referred to as red blood cells. Red blood cells are tasked with the oxygen exchange with other cells in the body. Red blood cells are anucleate (without a nucleus) and are much leaner than other cells in the sense that they lack many of the organelles found in other cells. They accomplish the gas transfer with the assistance of **hemoglobin**, an iron rich protein. Red blood cells are very numerous in the blood.

Less numerous, but equally important are **leukocytes**, or white blood cells. White blood cells are unique due to the fact that they are the

plasma
fluid portion of blood in which clotting elements and formed elements are suspended

albumin
a grouping of certain proteins such as those found in blood or egg whites

clotting factors
specific proteins that act together in clotting; defects in specific protein changes result in clotting conditions such as hemophilia

antibodies
component of the immune system that neutralizes antigens, encouraging long term immunity to the antigen

electrolytes
ions required by cells to regulate the electric charge and flow of water molecules across the cell membrane

formed elements
red or white blood cells or platelets separated from the fluid part of the blood

erythrocytes
red blood cells

hemoglobin
respiratory protein found in red blood cells, which aids in transportation of oxygen from lungs to tissues

leukocytes
white blood cells

Table 4–1   Facts About Blood

Blood is considered to have solid, liquid, and gaseous properties.

Our bodies produce 17 million red blood cells per second to replace the ones destroyed.

The body has about six quarts of blood. The blood travels through the body three times every minute. In one day, the blood travels four times the distance across the continental United States from coast to coast.

The weight of our complete blood supply is roughly 10 percent of our total body weight.

The heart pumps about 1 million barrels of blood during an average lifetime—that is enough to fill more than three supertankers.

Blood is classified as a circulating connective tissue.

Oxygenated blood is a brighter and purer red compared to the duller deoxygenated load carried by the veins.

Blood temperature and flow is regulated by a delicate balance called homeostasis. Blood temperature is maintained at 100.4° Fahrenheit, slightly warmer than overall body temperature.

White blood cells are bigger than and different in appearance from red blood cells. White cells circulate in the blood, but they can also change their shape to squeeze through a capillary and digest germs.

When blood becomes too cold, it is called "hypothermia." When blood flow is temporarily cut off then releases, it is called "restriction." If blood gets too warm, it is called "hyperthermia." All of these conditions have severe consequences ranging from tissue necrosis to death.

Flow restriction, hypothermia, and hyperthermia are also used as therapies for massage, cancer, and brain injuries, respectively.

---

only complete cells found in the blood (complete with nucleus, mitochondria, and other common organelles). White blood cells play an important role in protecting the body against disease and infection. Unlike red blood cells, white blood cells can exit and reenter the bloodstream at will. To this avail, white blood cells use the flow of blood as a transport mechanism to wherever in the body they are needed. Through a complex communication system, at the first sign of infection, the body increases leukocyte production and dispatches them for damage control.

There are two subcategories of leukocytes, **granulocytes** and **agranulocytes**. Granulocytes have granules, and they are highly specialized **phagocytes**. Agranulocytes are more general phagocytes and play

granulocytes
type of white blood cells containing granules

agranulocytes
nongranular white blood cells

phagocytes
waste clearing white blood cells

Table 4–2 Plasma Contents Carried in Blood

Substance	Function
Water	Transports minerals and formed elements; retains heat
Albumin	Transports fatty acids, hormones, drugs; maintains osmotic pressure; and buffers pH
Clotting factors	Essential to wound healing and tissue continuity
Antibodies	Proteins dispatched by the immune system to identify and neutralize foreign bodies
Electrolytes	Trace minerals that assist osmotic pressure and aid hydration of muscles and nerves
Nutrients	Vitamins, amino acids, and fatty acids essential to tissues and organs
Waste products	Lactic acid, urea, uric acid
Respiratory gases	Oxygen and carbon dioxide
Hormones	Vital to intercellular communication

Table 4–3 Formed Elements Found in Blood

Erythrocytes (red blood cells)–anucleate cells that transport oxygen to other cells by way of hemoglobin

Leukocytes (white blood cells)–specialized cells that work with the immune system to combat disease and infection; less numerous than erythrocytes

–Granulocytes	**Neutrophils**	Phagocytic cells that multiply at times of acute infection
	Eosinophils	Antiparasitic phagocytes
	Basophils	Provide histamine at inflammatory sites
–Agranulocytes	**Lymphocytes**	Produce antibodies and fight viral infections
	Monocytes	Phagocytes that become macrophages to aid overall systemic waste removal
	Platelets–required for blood clotting	

neutrophils
phagocytic white blood cells

eosinophils
type of granulated white blood cell

basophils
granulated white blood cell

lymphocytes
colorless cells found in blood and tissue that work toward cellular immunity

monocytes
large white blood cells that roam the blood stream neutralizing pathogens

platelets
a clotting element

an important role in the cellular cleanup. They work directly with the immune system as well as the lymphatic system.

Blood Disorders

With all that blood must accomplish in a quick trip throughout the body, any disturbance in its delicate balance can rapidly progress to a dire situation. With so many components, there are an equal number of disorders.

Anemia

Anemia is a common blood disorder that occurs when there are fewer red blood cells than normal, or there is a low concentration of hemoglobin in the blood. (See Table 4–4.) Most symptoms of anemia are a result of the decrease of oxygen in the cells or **hypoxia**. Because red blood cells carry oxygen via hemoglobin, a decreased production or number of these cells results in hypoxia. Many of the symptoms will not be present with mild anemia, as the body can often compensate for gradual changes in hemoglobin. There are several different subtypes of anemia. They include sickle-cell anemia, aplastic anemia, and hemolytic anemia.

anemia
condition characterized by a deficiency in iron, which is responsible for transporting oxygen in the blood

hypoxia
deficiency in the blood's ability to transport oxygen

Table 4–4   Symptoms of Anemia[1]
Abnormal paleness or lack of color of the skin
Increased heart rate (tachycardia)
Breathlessness or difficulty catching a breath (dyspnea)
Lack of energy or tiring easily (fatigue)
Dizziness or vertigo especially when standing
Headache
Irritability
Irregular menstrual cycles
Absent or delayed menstruation (amenorrhea)
Sore or swollen tongue (glossitis)
Jaundice or yellowing of skin, eyes, and mouth
Enlarged spleen or liver (splenomegaly, hepatomegaly)
Slow or delayed growth and development
Impaired wound and tissue healing

Thalassemia

Thalassemia is an inherited disorder that affects the production of normal hemoglobin (a type of protein in red blood cells that carries oxygen to the tissues in the body). Thalassemia includes a number of different forms of anemia. The severity and type of anemia depends upon the number of genes that are affected.

This disorder is common in populations around the Mediterranean Sea, Africa, and Southeast Asia. The presenting signs and symptoms of all forms of thalassemia point to anemia (a deficiency of red blood cells) in varying degrees from mild to severe.

Hemophilia

Hemophilia is an inherited bleeding disorder characterized by a reduced number or complete absence of clotting factors. The result is an inability to stop bleeding at the site of a wound, easy bruising, and bleeding from joints. It is a disease that is more common in men than women. There are a variety of subsets of this disorder that are determined by the specific clotting factor that is absent.

Leukemia

Leukemia is cancer of the blood that develops in the bone marrow. The bone marrow is the soft, spongy center of the long bones that produces the three major blood cells: white blood cells to fight infection, red blood cells that carry oxygen, and platelets that help with blood clotting and stopping bleeding. When a person has leukemia, the bone marrow, for an unknown reason, begins to make white blood cells that do not mature correctly, but continue to reproduce themselves. Normal, healthy cells reproduce only when there is enough space for them to fit. The body can regulate the production of cells by sending signals to stop reproduction. With leukemia, these cells do not respond to the signals to stop and thus reproduce, regardless of space available.

thalassemia
condition characterized by defective hemoglobin cells, resulting in oxygen deficiency

hemophilia
disorder characterized by deficiencies of clotting factors reducing the blood's ability to clot

leukemia
disease of the bone marrow characterized by excessive and unwanted white blood cell proliferation

■ THE HEART

Our individual hearts are roughly the size of our clenched fists. One might not expect that something so small can handle such copious responsibilities. Yet from the time we are just a few weeks old in our mothers' wombs, the heart manages its responsibilities with clock-like diligence. Literally, our hearts pump sustenance to every cell in our bodies. (See Figure 4–1.)

Located just left of center of the middle thorax cavity, the heart is surrounded by the lungs on each side and the diaphragm below. The

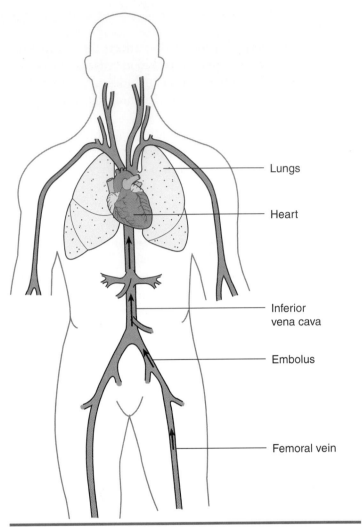

Figure 4–1 The heart is about the size of a clenched fist

pericardium
fluid-filled encasement surrounding the heart and major blood vessels

epicardium
inner layer of the pericardium that has direct contact with the heart

myocardium
muscular tissue around the heart

exterior of the heart is surrounded by a thin fibrous sheath called the **pericardium** and is attached to surrounding organs by the **epicardium**. The pericardium blends in with walls of the heart and actually forms the outermost layer of three of the walls. The second layer, the **myocardium**, is muscle tissue that contracts, which results in "pumping" blood through the chambers and throughout the body. The innermost layer of the heart, the endocardium, is made up of serous epithelial tissue. This tissue blends in with the connecting blood vessels, enabling the critical fluid transfers.

The heart's contractions occur independently of the nervous system. This means that unlike most muscles, which move in response to cues from the nerves connected to the brain, the heart contracts automatically.

The cells within the heart contract on their own with the help of specialized tissue that is a hybrid of muscle and nervous tissue. This hybrid tissue is found nowhere else in the body. The heart's contractions form what we hear as our heartbeat. We hear the left ventricle, which does the majority of the pumping, when listening through a **stethoscope**. Our **blood pressure** is decided by the contraction (**systole**) and relaxation (**diastole**) of the heart. The cardiac cycle is the process of both atria relaxing and contracting. Typically, this occurs 75 times a minute in a healthy adult.[2]

Although the heart is basically hollow, it contains divided sections called chambers. This prevents the blood that has been **oxygenated** from interacting with blood that has lost its oxygen load.

The Chambers of the Heart

Within the heart, there exist four chambers, two on the top and two on the bottom. The two chambers on top are called **atria** (atrium in the singular), and they receive blood. The two bottom chambers are called **ventricles**, and they pump blood.

The right atrium receives blood from the rest of the body, and the left atrium receives blood from lungs. The difference between the blood they receive is the presence or lack of oxygen. The right atrium receives blood that is deoxygenated from the body and sends it to the right ventricle, from which it is pumped to the lungs to pick up another load of oxygen. This is referred to as **pulmonary circulation**. The left atrium receives oxygenated blood from the lungs and sends it to the left ventricle, from which it is pumped into the body. This is referred to as **systemic circulation**. Because the oxygen-rich blood pumped out to the body from the left ventricle has to travel such a great distance, its walls are much thicker. (See Figure 4–2.)

The two chambers on top are called atria, and they receive blood. The two bottom chambers are called ventricles, and they pump blood.

Aiding the pumping processes of the heart are valves, which prevent the backflow of blood between chambers. On the left side, the valve that prevents backflow is called the **bicuspid valve**. It is composed of a dual layer of endocardium tissue. Likewise, separating the right chambers is the **tricuspid valve**. The tricuspid is made up of three layers of endocardium tissue. Collectively, these two valves are referred to as AV valves, or **atrioventricular valves**. The second set of valves is called the **semilunar valves**. These valves regulate the flow of blood between the ventricles and the major blood vessel to which they connect. On the right side is the **pulmonary valve**, and on the left side is the **aortic semilunar valve**. Without the work of these valves, our hearts would not function optimally.

stethoscope
device used to magnify the sound of a beating heart

blood pressure
the tension against the arterial walls, read in contraction and relaxation

systole
part of the normal rhythmic heartbeat during which the filled ventricles pump blood out the pulmonary artery and the aorta

diastole
part of the normal rhythm of the heart during which the heart chambers fill with blood

oxygenated
rich in oxygen

atria
the two upper chambers of the heart receive blood for reoxygenation

ventricles
the lower chambers of the heart, which force blood either to the lungs for oxygenation or out to the body

pulmonary circulation
path deoxygenated blood takes to become oxygenated; in through the right ventricle, into the lungs through the pulmonary artery, and into the left atrium via the pulmonary vein

systemic circulation
blood and lymph circulation from the heart, through the arteries, to tissue and cells, and back to the heart by way of the veins

bicuspid valve
heart valve located between the left atrium and ventricle that regulates backflow between the two chambers

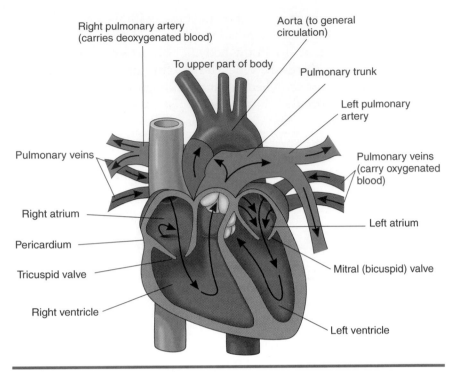

Figure 4–2 Inside the heart, there are four chambers, two on top and two on the bottom

tricuspid valve
heart valve that prevents backflow between the right atrium and right ventricle

atrioventricular valves
trio of valves that prevent blood flow back into the ventricles of the heart

semilunar valves
valves of the arteries, preventing backflow from arteries into the ventricles

pulmonary valve
valve that separates the pulmonary path from the right ventricle

aortic semilunar valve
trio of valves that prevent blood flow back into the heart

heart disease
any condition that impairs the normal function of the heart and/or blood vessels

■ HEART DISEASE

Heart disease is the broad term used to describe any condition that affects the performance of the heart or the cardiovascular system. As a whole, heart disease is the leading cause of death among both American men and women.

As we age, normal wear and tear occurs in the cardiovascular system. In particular, the arteries lose elasticity with time. However, the cardiovascular system is resilient and reliable. Most of the conditions that qualify as heart disease (barring congenital conditions) have a manageable environmental component. Medical professionals agree that diet, exercise, and elimination of excesses (such as smoking and drinking) can reduce heart disease. (See Table 4–5.)

■ THE ARTERIAL SYSTEM

As mentioned above, arteries supply the body with oxygenated blood pumped out from the left ventricle. (See Figure 4–3.) While this sounds

Table 4–5	Heart Diseases
Condition	**Description**
Coronary Artery Disease (CAD)	Plaque caused by fat clogs the arteries, restricting oxygen and nutrients needed by the heart; often results in a heart attack
Arrythmia	Heart rate either lower than normal (<60 bpm) or higher than normal (>100 bpm)
Heart Failure	Reduction in the pumping ability of the heart resulting in limited flow (congestion)
Heart Valve Disease	Inefficacy of valves in the heart resulting in backflow or limited flow; often congenital
Congenital Heart Conditions	A defect in one of the heart's structures that occurs prior to birth
Cardiomyopathy	Gradual enlarging of heart tissues resulting in heart failure
Pericarditis	Inflammation of the pericardium
Aortic Aneurism	Weakened pocket of lining in the aorta

simple, the actual process is quite complicated. In fact, the breadth of this discussion is much greater than the scope of this book. However, for the treatments that you, an aspiring aesthetician, will be performing, it is important to have a working knowledge of the arterial system.

The arterial system is the higher pressure portion of the circulatory system. Once the heart pumps the blood through the aorta and the greater arteries, the blood branches out through the lesser arterial structures and feeds oxygen to cells and organs. Without this, our cells would die, as would we.

The Arteries

When you consider the arteries of your body, think of a tree that starts from a trunk and divides into branches, and continues to divide into ever smaller twigs. In this case, the trunk starts from the left ventricle, which pumps oxygenated blood. The trunk is formed by the **aorta**, and the branches and twigs forming the arterial system reach to every part of the body and its organs, with these exceptions: hair, nails, epidermis (top layer of skin), cartilage, and cornea. The larger trunks of the arterial system tend to be in places more protected from harm, running in the limbs

aorta
primary artery that carries blood from the heart to the auxiliary arteries of the trunk and limbs

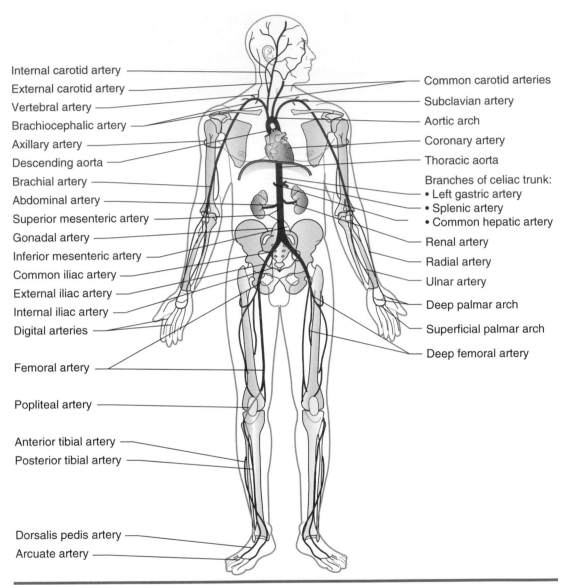

Internal carotid artery

External carotid artery

Vertebral artery

Brachiocephalic artery

Axillary artery

Descending aorta

Brachial artery

Abdominal artery

Superior mesenteric artery

Gonadal artery

Inferior mesenteric artery

Common iliac artery

External iliac artery

Internal iliac artery

Digital arteries

Femoral artery

Popliteal artery

Anterior tibial artery

Posterior tibial artery

Dorsalis pedis artery

Arcuate artery

Common carotid arteries

Subclavian artery

Aortic arch

Coronary artery

Thoracic aorta

Branches of celiac trunk:
• Left gastric artery
• Splenic artery
• Common hepatic artery

Renal artery

Radial artery

Ulnar artery

Deep palmar arch

Superficial palmar arch

Deep femoral artery

Figure 4–3 Arteries supply oxygenated blood to the body, which is pumped from the left ventricle

flexor
the major muscle or muscle group that causes flexation

anastomosis
the connection point of different parts of a branching network

through the **flexor** or contractile surfaces. This protects the body from fatal injury if a minor laceration or wound occurs.

Arteries are tubular, and as they distribute themselves they communicate with each other in what are called anastomoses (singular form is **anastomosis**). Intertwine your fingers and you are envisioning anastomosis. Anastomoses enable blood to reach areas that need it, such as the brain, in great concentration. Another area that needs a lot of oxygenated blood is the abdomen, so that we may digest our food. The intestinal arteries have numerous anastomoses between and among their larger arterial branches. In our limbs, the largest and most numerous anastomoses occur around the joints, where branches of an artery above may unite with branches of an artery below. Anastomoses around joints are of interest to surgeons. This is because when a **ligature** of a vessel occurs in a surgical procedure the anastomoses may enlarge to produce **collateral circulation** around the tied-off place.

The arteries' duty is to deliver blood quickly, and in most places the vessels flow in fairly straight lines. There are occasions, however, when it is to their benefit for them to become **tortuous**, or highly curved and bent. This happens with the external maxillary artery, which serves much of the face, and with the labial arteries of the lips—these arteries become quite tortuous to accommodate the variety of facial movements of which we and other primates are capable. The uterine arteries are tortuous as well, because during pregnancy they need to accommodate a growing fetus.

ligature
a tying or other binding mechanism

collateral circulation
additional circulation, side by side

tortuous
taking a twisting, nonlinear path

capillaries
tiny blood vessels that connect arterioles and venules, and where gases and other substances are exchanged

Arterioles

If arteries are the trunk of the tree, then arterioles are the branches. These smaller arterial routes connect to organs and other tissues, and eventually feed the capillaries. Arterioles have the greatest collective influence on both local blood flow and on overall blood pressure. They are the primary "adjustable nozzles" in the blood system, across which the greatest pressure drop occurs. The combination of heart output (cardiac output) and total peripheral resistance, which refers to the collective resistance of all of the body's arterioles, are the principal determinants of arterial blood pressure at any given moment.

Capillaries

If arteries are the trunk and arterioles are branches, then **capillaries** are the leaves. (See Figure 4–4.) They are the smallest part of the network, and it is here that they connect with the venous system to begin their journey back to the heart. Within capillaries, all the true action of the circulatory system occurs. This is where gases and nutrients are exchanged and wastes are eliminated.

The Venous System

The venous system is a complex network of veins and venules that are tasked with returning blood to the heart and lungs for a recharge of

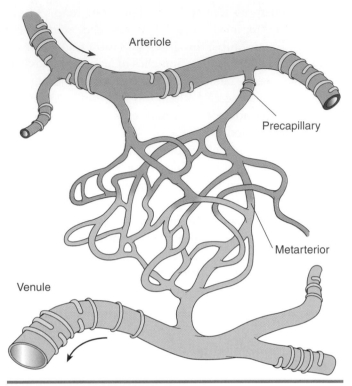

Figure 4–4 Capillaries are the smallest part of the circulatory network

oxygen. The venous system picks up where the arterial system leaves off, with the capillaries. (See Figure 4–5.)

The Veins

As you are by now aware, veins convey **deoxygenated** blood from various parts of the body back to the heart. Veins arise from tiny **plexuses** or networks of intersecting venules, which receive blood from capillaries, tiny branches of arterioles. As these venous branches travel, they unite with each other into trunks, coursing along and constantly receiving tributaries or joining other veins. As they approach the heart, the veins increase in size to the point of being larger than corresponding arteries. (See Figure 4–6.)

You might not suspect this, but veins are not only larger than arteries, veins are also more numerous. Therefore, the capacity of the venous system to hold its product—blood—is greater than that of the arterial system. We will discuss this concept more in the following section when we discuss peripheral venous return.

deoxygenated
formerly oxygen rich blood whose nutrient load has been distributed and is routed back to the heart, via the veins, for oxygenation

plexuses
a network of blood vessels

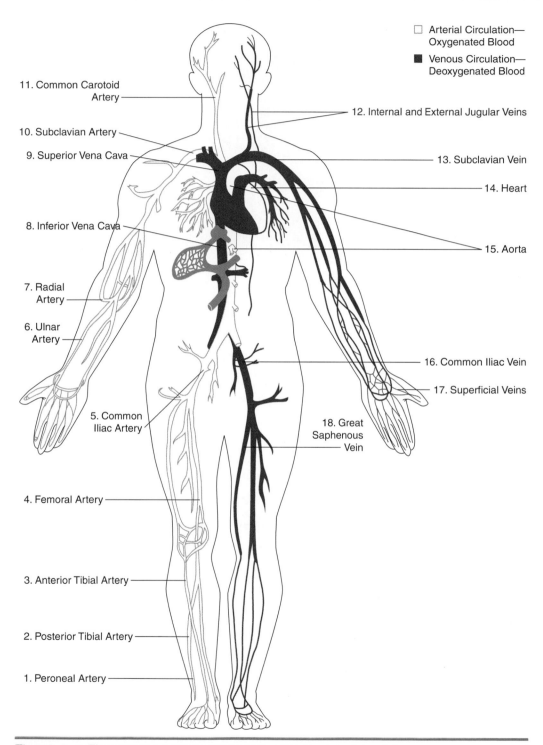

☐ Arterial Circulation—
  Oxygenated Blood

■ Venous Circulation—
  Deoxygenated Blood

11. Common Carotoid Artery

10. Subclavian Artery

9. Superior Vena Cava

8. Inferior Vena Cava

7. Radial Artery

6. Ulnar Artery

5. Common Iliac Artery

4. Femoral Artery

3. Anterior Tibial Artery

2. Posterior Tibial Artery

1. Peroneal Artery

12. Internal and External Jugular Veins

13. Subclavian Vein

14. Heart

15. Aorta

16. Common Iliac Vein

17. Superficial Veins

18. Great Saphenous Vein

Figure 4–5 The venous system returns blood to the heart, to pick up more oxygen and nutrients

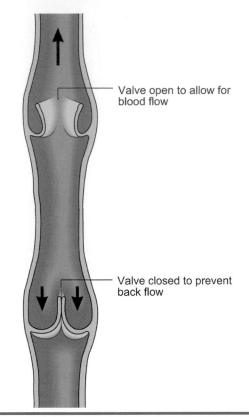

Blood flow toward the heart

Valve open to allow for
blood flow

Valve closed to prevent
back flow

Figure 4–6 Veins have valves inside the vessel
that open and close to assist blood flow back to
the heart

cylindrical
circular

Like arteries, veins are **cylindrical** in shape, but, unlike arteries, their
walls are thin and collapse when they are empty. Like arteries, veins communicate freely with one another and particularly in those areas of the
body that require more blood removal. Large and frequent anastomoses
exist between veins in your neck, where a blockage of blood returning
from the brain would be unacceptable. Veins also compose many plexuses
in the abdominal and pelvic region, particularly in spermatic and uterine
regions. (See Figure 4–7.)

Peripheral Venous Return

The circulatory system is a closed circuit system, which means that the
blood flow leaving the extremities via the veins must equal that being
pumped in via the arteries. The flow is variable, dependant upon such
factors as temperature, degree of activity, and positioning.

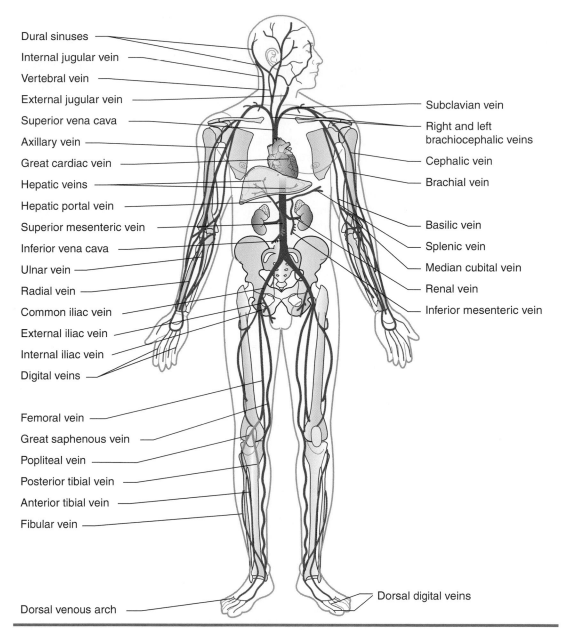

Dural sinuses

Internal jugular vein

Vertebral vein

External jugular vein

Superior vena cava

Axillary vein

Great cardiac vein

Hepatic veins

Hepatic portal vein

Superior mesenteric vein

Inferior vena cava

Ulnar vein

Radial vein

Common iliac vein

External iliac vein

Internal iliac vein

Digital veins

Femoral vein

Great saphenous vein

Popliteal vein

Posterior tibial vein

Anterior tibial vein

Fibular vein

Dorsal venous arch

Subclavian vein

Right and left brachiocephalic veins

Cephalic vein

Brachial vein

Basilic vein

Splenic vein

Median cubital vein

Renal vein

Inferior mesenteric vein

Dorsal digital veins

Figure 4–7 The circulatory system is a closed circuit system of arteries, veins, capillaries, and, of course, the heart

There are many diseases that present with **peripheral edema**; among them are congestive heart failure, kidney failure, stasis dermatitis, and varicose veins. Each has its origins in a different body system, but they all cause a phenomenon known as edema.

peripheral edema
swelling resulting from fluid accumulation in the lower limbs

When healthy individuals are standing or sitting, as they are most of the waking hours, the circulatory system is forced to work against the forces of gravity. To accomplish this, deep veins use the muscle and tendons surrounding them to act as a pump to assist the blood's ultimate return to the heart. This is accomplished mostly by the calves, with the help of the valves. Almost all of the peripheral venous return is done by the calves. However, the foot and ankle also contribute. This explains why walking is so good for the circulation of blood.

Hydrostatic pressure is caused by the weight of the fluid, in this case blood, in the veins.

Hydrostatic pressure may be caused by obesity and pregnancy, which can cause pressure on the pelvic veins, pushing the blood backwards, causing injury to the valves.

■ DISEASED VEINS

In the section above, you learned that occasional constrictions or visual irregularities in the surface of veins indicate the presence of valves. The purpose of venous valves is much the same as valves along a water pipe: to prevent backflow. Valves are more numerous in deep veins than in superficial veins, and, because we are upright creatures, valves are also more common in veins of the lower limb than in those of the upper.

When blood is returning to the heart, it is generally flowing upward against gravity. The valves in the veins reduce the pressure of blood below by supporting it at different places on its way up. Unlike deep veins, veins near the surface of the skin are not supported by muscles and so they get no assistance in the task of keeping blood flowing upward.

When valves in our legs get "leaky" and no longer do their job of preventing backflow, they are said to have become "incompetent." Incompetent valves allow gravity to pull blood back down into ever-widening pools in the veins, creating hydrostatic pressure. The vein begins to bulge and stretch, and we have all seen the results: varicose veins and spider veins.

What causes **varicose veins** and spider veins is hard to say with certainty, but they can be associated with pregnancy, hormonal shifts, weight gain, standing occupations, and certain medications, as well as certain other conditions. Pregnancy is a particular culprit: not only does it increase hormone levels and blood volume, which causes veins to enlarge, but the enlarged uterus also increases pressure on the veins. Successive pregnancies may make the problem worse. Certain medical conditions such as diabetes affect blood flow and may dispose a person to varicose veins. Finally, we cannot discount simple heredity, which may be the

hydrostatic pressure
means of devising fluid pressure by means of measuring the pressure imposed by an external force

varicose veins
condition characterized by swollen veins, most commonly in the legs

chief contributor to spider and varicose veins. Like all aspects of aging, those physiologic attributes that you recall from your parents may be yours as well in the aging process.

Although the vast majority of varicose and incompetent veins are merely inconvenient, many are painful and some may indicate the presence of disease; think peripheral vascular edema. If your client who complains of pain has not had this condition evaluated by a physician, tell him or her that it might be a symptom of something more serious and urge him or her to do so.

Varicose Veins

The differences between varicose veins and spider veins are primarily size and depth. Varicose veins are larger and generally deeper than spider veins. (See Figure 4–8.) Varicose veins can also be found in internal organs; for example, hemorrhoids are varicose veins around the anus.

Varicose veins in the legs may measure more than a quarter inch across and tend to bulge as blood backs up behind incompetent valves. When blood congestion is regular, the veins enlarge and distend, causing them to be not only more prominent but, in some cases, uncomfortable. In some cases, simple sclerotherapy is sufficient to deal with varicose veins, but other options are also available.

The Lymphatic System

Our lymphatic system is a vital component to both our circulatory system and our immune system. Often overlooked, its functions are vital to our survival. The main purpose of the lymphatic system is basically that of cleanup for the circulatory system. As mentioned, arteries and veins make their fluid, gas, and nutrient exchanges with our bodies by way of capillaries and venules, respectively. This process is far from seamless. Excess fluid, called **lymph**, seeps out and must be reabsorbed in order for blood levels to remain at acceptable levels to perform its varied duties. This is where the lymphatic system comes in. (See Figure 4–9.)

Without **lymphatic vessels** and organs, fluid would accumulate, resulting in swelling and redness, a condition we refer to as **edema**. Lymphatic vessels reabsorb the lymph, store it in the lymphatic collecting vessels and lymph nodes, and return it to the heart. Unlike capillaries and venules, lymphatic vessels are highly permeable. To this effect, bacteria, viruses, and cell debris can easily find their way inside. If not for the lymph nodes, this means of entry could be catastrophic. The **lymph nodes**, scattered throughout the body, remove all the excess debris while the remaining fluid undergoes a quality control check with the

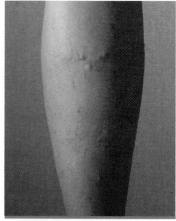

Figure 4–8 Incompetent veins have valves that are no longer working properly, these larger veins become diseased and are called varicosed

lymph
waste clearing fluid that contains white blood cells and lymphocytes to the blood for future waste removal

lymphatic vessels
tubes through which lymph flows through its network

edema
swelling resulting from excessive fluid buildup in tissue

lymph nodes
small glands that store the wastes collected by lymphocytes

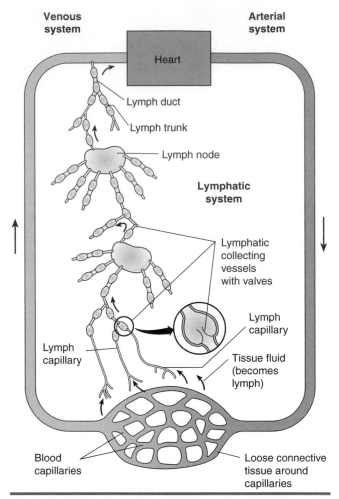

Figure 4–9 The lymph system runs alongside the circulatory system and removes bacteria, cell debris, and viruses from the body

help of the immune system. Once cleared for reentry, lymph returns to the bloodstream by way of the thoracic duct. There, it connects to the subclavian vein, where it returns to the heart for a re-up of nutrients.

Lymphatic Drainage

As vital to our survival as the lymphatic system is, it is prone to fatigue overtime, resulting in fluid stagnation. This stagnation results in edema, and has consequences for the circulatory system, immune system, and nervous system. To combat this, **lymphatic drainage** is often employed to manually rouse the system to a greater level of efficacy.

lymphatic drainage
technique of manually flushing clogged lymphatic vessels and glands

Table 4–6   Benefits from Lymphatic Drainage
Reduces edema
Detoxifies
Enhances tissue regeneration
Combats aging
Relieves certain inflammations
Relieves pain
Combats fatigue
Relieves constipation
Promotes relaxation

Lymphatic drainage was first employed by a European doctor, Dr. E. Vodder, in the 1930s. His methods were then built upon with the exacting science of Dr. Bruno Chikly. Using precise anatomy and specific manual processes, practitioners detect the direction and quality of lymphatic flow, and manually encourage optimal flow by means of alternate pathways. In doing so, researchers believe that the resulting optimal flow stimulates the overall circulation, stimulates immunologic protection, and promotes optimal nervous system function. (See Table 4–6.)

Conclusion

At the center of the circulatory system is the heart. But, as we have learned, the heart alone is not responsible for the cardiovascular system. The arteries, veins, lymph system, and heart work to transport blood to the tissues. Any disease that affects a part of the system, may, in fact, affect the functioning of the entire system. It is important to counsel our patients to a healthy life-style to sustain good cardiac health. This would include attention to diet and exercise.

⫸ ⟩ ⟩ TOP 10 TIPS TO TAKE TO THE CLINIC

1. Lymphatic drainage can be beneficial to the postsurgical patient.
2. Varicose veins are due to incompetent valves.
3. Arteries branch out into smaller and smaller vessels, called arterioles.

4. Capillaries connect arterioles to venules.

5. The body has six quarts of blood.

6. Lack of energy can be a sign of anemia.

7. Peripheral edema can be a sign of a serious disease.

8. The veins carry deoxygenated blood.

9. The arteries carry oxygenated blood.

10. The heart is the center of the circulatory system.

CHAPTER QUESTIONS

1. What is lymphatic drainage?

2. Name the parts of the circulatory system.

3. How are veins different from arteries?

4. How do varicose veins occur?

5. Name two heart diseases.

CHAPTER REFERENCES

1. http://uuhsc.utah.edu/
2. Marieb, E. N. (2006). *Essentials of Human Anatomy & Physiology* (8th ed.). San Francisco, CA: Pearson Education.

BIBLIOGRAPHY

American College of Phlebology. Available at http://www.phlebology.org/

American Society of Plastic Surgeons. *Sclerotherapy*. Available at http://www.plasticsurgery.org

Chikly, B. (1996). *Lymphatic Drainage Therapy*. Available at http://www.arthritistrust.org

Gray's Anatomy Online, 2000. Available at http://education.yahoo.com/

International Alliance of Healthcare Educators. *Lymphatic Drainage Therapy*. Available at http://www.iahe.com

Marieb, E. N. (2006). *Essentials of Human Anatomy & Physiology* (8th ed.). San Francisco, CA: Pearson Education.

Medlineplus.com. (2005, September 16). *Medical Encyclopedia: Foot, Leg, and Ankle Swelling*. Available at http://www.nlm.nih.gov/

Medlineplus.com. (2005, September 16). *Medical Encyclopedia: Lower Leg Edema*. Available at http://www.nlm.nih.gov/

Medlineplus.com. (2005, September 16). *Medical Encyclopedia: Venous Insufficiency*. Available at http://www.nlm.nih.gov/

NHS Direct Online Health Encyclopedia. Available at http://www.nhsdirect.nhs.uk

Body Wraps and Masks

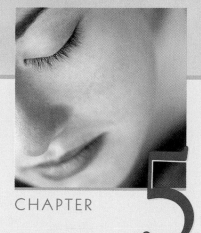

CHAPTER 5

KEY TERMS

aromatherapy	elastic wraps	prone position
blanket wraps	herb wraps	Scotch hose
body wrap	hydrocollators	seaweed wraps
cellophane body wrap	Kneipp Body Wraps	supine position
confidentiality	occlusion	thalassotherapy
contraindications	patchouli	treatment table
diaphoretic		

LEARNING OBJECTIVES

After completing this chapter, you should be able to:

1. Discuss body wraps and masks.
2. Discuss table options and client preparation.
3. Discuss confidentiality and privacy issues.
4. Discuss types of wraps and mask options.
5. Discuss the supplies and equipment needed for spa treatments.

INTRODUCTION

Having explained some of the more fundamental aspects of **body wrap** stimulation, it is time to delve a bit deeper and explain the treatment itself. A body treatment is simply a facial for the body. Though the concerns that body wraps and facials address may differ (i.e., rejuvenation versus cellulite), there are many similarities between the two. Some basic commonalities shared between the two include cleansing, exfoliation, targeted skin treatments, and metabolic stimulation.[1] In addition, body treatments offer many additional benefits, such as hydration, detoxification, and relaxation. Certain specific treatments may also reduce the appearance of cellulite or sun damage.

While there is a certain amount of debate as to the efficacy of body wraps to produce long term results for certain goals (i.e., cellulite reduction), it is well known that body wraps are a superb means of promoting healthy skin all over the body. Not to mention, they are an excellent means of pampering and achieving a state of relaxation. (See Figure 5–1.) As an aesthetician, it will be your goal to assist your clients in achieving their skin care goals. Body wraps are one such means of doing so.

body wrap
a spa treatment that uses blankets, cellophane, or other products

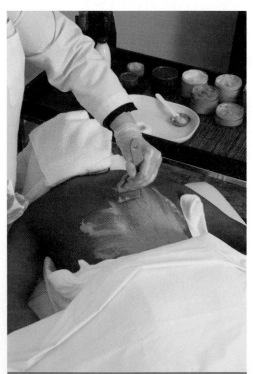

Figure 5–1 A body treatment is simply a facial for the body

Let us take the process apart and examine the basics, starting with equipment.

Treatment Table Options

One of the most important pieces of professional equipment you will use as an aesthetician is the **treatment table**. This piece of equipment is especially vital for performing body wraps. Treatment tables need to be durable, functional, and comfortable for both your client and you. (See Figure 5–2.)

There is a wide variety of treatment table options. If you are doing body treatments, you may want to consider a table that has a cutout for the client's face when he or she is lying in the **prone position**. Most procedure chairs found in spas do not provide such modifications. In chairs without cutouts, clients may be uncomfortable lying with their heads turned to the side for extended periods of time. Since one of the foremost goals with body wraps is to achieve a relaxed state, such a position would be juxtaposed to our intent. Therefore, you might want to consider a massage table for performing body wraps. In addition to being comfortable for the client, the massage table also offers the ability to adjust the height of the table to ensure comfort for the technician as well. Some manufacturers offer a hydraulic table that is easily adjusted.

Some spas or clinics have a wet room. If your facility has a wet room, your table options expand. Waterproof treatment tables are modified versions of a massage table that have waterproof legs and a more durable material to cover the top where water would otherwise damage a standard table. Other options include wet tables, which are composed of a composite or plastic material as the base and have a waterproof removable pad. These tables are often found where spa treatment showers or hoses are used.

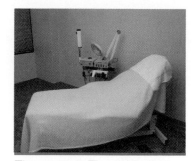

Figure 5–2 The table that you choose should be durable, functional, and comfortable for both your client and you

treatment table
the table specifically designed to aid in offering treatments such as facials, body wraps, or massages

prone position
lying with the front or face downward

confidentiality
prohibits you from disclosing information about the client's treatment or chart to others and requires that you take precautions with the information to ensure that only authorized access occurs

Confidentiality and Privacy

Confidentiality should be one of the core tenets of your facility and practice. As with any treatment, your clients should feel that all their information is handled with safeguards to ensure confidentiality. This means that all personal information is to be safeguarded and withheld from individuals who are not involved with the treatment plan. All personal information, including names, should be kept in a safe place and not discussed in the presence of nonessential staff and other clients.

By respecting their privacy and creating a trusting environment, you are promoting an open and comfortable environment in which your clients will feel safe and respected. It is important that your clients feel comfortable disclosing even the most personal information with you as it may affect the outcome of or candidacy for treatment. Even the smallest plastic surgery procedure, application of a filler, or injectable can be contraindicative to the treatment's results.

In the course of providing spa services to your client, you will find yourself exchanging information about your client with other aestheticians or spa personnel. These discussions are often necessary for client care and are an integral part of ensuring the optimal outcome of the treatment. Your disclosure is justifiable as long as you take precautions to limit the ability of others to hear or see confidential charts and information. Discussing a client's information in a public place or with other clients is prohibited.

There are two exceptions when a client's private information can be disclosed. The first is if you can protect the identifiable individuals from any serious threat of harm, as in the case of abuse or domestic violence. In this case you have a duty to disclose the information to the proper authorities. The second exception is if you are required by state law to report certain communicable/infectious diseases to public health authorities.

Health Screening, Indications, and Contraindications

As with any aesthetic service, you want to assess the suitability of your client's treatment. When applying products to large areas or to the entire body, the risk for allergies and the complications associated with the allergic response and **contraindications** increases substantially. For this reason, it is important to be especially thorough with all of your client intake and assessment forms. If you conduct a consultation prior to treatment, be certain that the client has completed all the necessary paperwork, including a thorough health history as well as a skin history. Make sure that they are complete. Go over the answers with the client and complete any portion left undone. Determine if the treatment is indicated and look for responses that might be contraindicated for the treatment. Follow up any concerns with the appropriate response (for instance, consulting with the supervising physician if one is on staff at your place of employment).

As with any treatment, there are specific contraindications provided by the manufacturer of the product, so it is important to review and update all forms every time a client returns to ensure that his or her health records remain current.[2]

■ PREPARING THE CLIENT

Always greet your client in a professional manner. Since body treatments require consideration of and thoughtfulness for a client's modesty, it is

contraindications
any service or activity that could cause harm to the client

A little more preparation is required for a body treatment than for a standard facial. Though the room's preparation is directly associated with the type of treatment your client receives, there are some fundamental preparation guidelines you should always follow.

General Contraindications for Facial Procedures

Clients who are under physician's care for skin disease.

Clients currently using prescription keratolytics: tretinoin (Retin-A or Renova), Azelaic Acid (Azelex), tazarotene (Tazorac), adapalene (different), or other procedures, drugs, or cosmetics that cause exfoliation.

Clients who are taking Accutane or clients who have used Accutane in the past six months.

Clients who have broken skin, visible redness, irritation or inflammation, fever blisters, cold sores, rosacea flare-ups, sunburn,

To prepare the treatment room, be sure it is extremely clean and sanitized. This will help put the client at ease. The table should be prepared with materials needed. Keep in mind that the outermost layer of material represents the first treatment that will be performed.

important that the first thing you accomplish is to put him or her at ease by demonstrating your professionalism.

As mentioned, it is extremely important to get a complete and thorough health history of your client. As the name implies, these treatments involve the whole body and therefore may pose a greater risk to the client based on his health history. By reviewing your client's health

General Contraindicative Conditions for Body Treatments

- Pregnancy
- Open wounds
- Varicose veins
- High/low blood pressure
- Medications for high or low blood pressure
- Heat sensitivity
- Heart problems
- Diabetes
- Lupus
- Raynaud's disease
- Chemotherapy
- Mastectomy or breast reduction
- Plastic surgery
- Pre- and postsurgery as indicated by physician
- Loss of sensitivity or numbness
- Allergies to products being used
- Claustrophobia

> ### *Treatment Room Preparation Guidelines*
>
> - Cover the table with a sheet.
> - Cover the table with a wool or insulating blanket.
> - Cover the table with a thermal blanket.
> - Cover the table with a plastic wrap sheet. (Depending on the treatment, you may want to cover this plastic sheet with a cotton one for comfort purposes.)
> - Provide an additional sheet or large towel for the client to slide under to maintain proper draping while implementing the procedure.
> - Provide two modesty towels for women and one for men if disposable undergarments are not worn.

history, you can ensure that the treatments performed will not be contraindicated with any existing medical conditions. Reviewing health history is not only important for your purposes, but it conveys to the client that you are concerned about his well-being, thus making him feel more comfortable. Avoid being too "medicinal" in your approach, as this may have the opposite effect. Be warm and compassionate in your interactions with your clients by promoting an atmosphere where they can truly relax. It is important to not promote conversations that are off topic but encourage the clients to feel comfortable enough to disclose any information that may affect the outcomes of their treatment.

Next, it is equally important to discuss modesty with your client. Advise the client of the steps you will be taking, and what is required from him or her. (See Figure 5–3.) Remind the client to be comfortable and ask if he or she has any concerns. Be open to any suggestion he or she may have that will not impede the treatment. Your goal is to make the client as comfortable as possible. Otherwise, the treatment might not have the desired results. Be sure to let the client know that you will keep the entire body draped except for the part that is being treated. Usually body treatments are performed on nude clients or those wearing disposable undergarments that are provided by the spa. Ask the client for a preference. While some people are very comfortable in the nude, others are very shy.

After establishing that it is safe to proceed with the treatment, help your client onto the table, keeping his or her comfort in mind. Situate the client on the table in a prone or **supine position**, according to the treatment. Plan ahead and allow his or her placement on the table for the least amount of movement by the client. Last, but not least, never leave a client unattended during a body treatment. Leaving someone unattended for

supine position
lying with the front or face upward

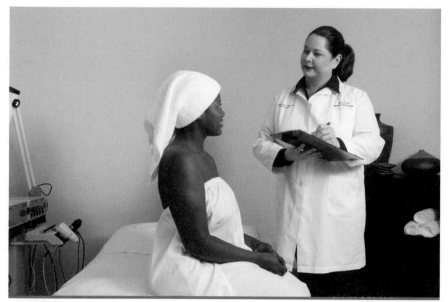

Figure 5–3 Aestheticians should discuss with the client the wrap options available

any amount of time can be dangerous, as problems need to be addressed quickly. If you have a client who is allergic to sulfur, commonly found in some body treatment masks, a simple spa treatment can result in anaphylaxis, a serious and rapid allergic reaction. If the reaction is severe enough and the affected person does not receive immediate medical attention, it can result in death.

Comfort

The key to the success of every treatment is relaxation. In order for the client to relax, he or she must be comfortable. During the relaxation response, breathing, metabolic heart rate, and blood pressure all slow down. The long term effects of regularly inducing this response include improved concentration and increased energy, and your body becomes less responsive to the stress hormones.[3] Quiet leads to relaxation. To keep noise to a minimum, be prepared for the treatment and perform your duties as quietly as possible, wearing soft-soled or rubber shoes. Avoid running water in the sink while the client is relaxing. Temperature is another component of relaxation. Some people have differing thresholds for temperature comfort, so be sure to ask if the temperature setting is appealing to the client. Other important comfort factors include lighting and sound. Your lighting should create a relaxing environment. Bright lighting can be annoying. Also avoid unnecessary conversation and keep surrounding sounds, such as doors slamming, garbage cans

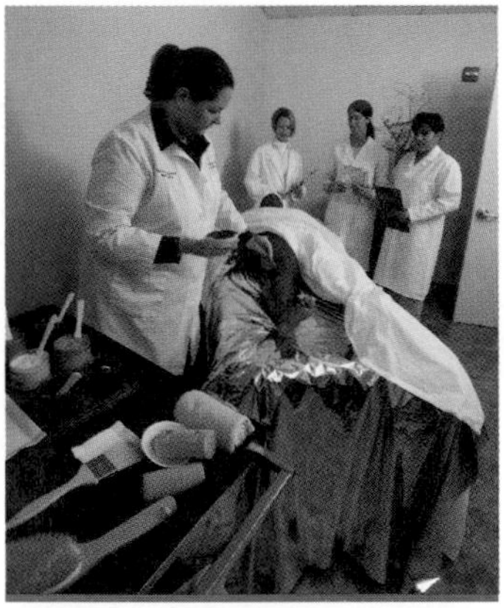

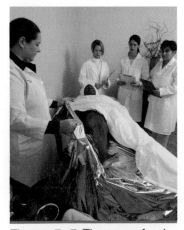

Figure 5–4 Application of a body mask

Figure 5–5 The use of cellophane to retain body heat during the processing phase of a body mask treatment

General Client Preparation Procedures

Once the treatment room is fully prepared, you may bring the client into it. At this point, you should focus on how to properly drape the client for service. Some general client preparation guidelines include the following:

- Give the client instructions before you leave the room. These instructions should include the removal of all jewelry. Have the client wear disposable undergarments or, if preferred, remove all clothing. Show the client the proper place to store all personal items.

- Instruct the client on how to get onto the treatment table and into position. Keep in mind this may be his or her first treatment, so be sure all of your instructions are clear and that your client understands them. This is also the time to show the client the additional sheet he or she can slide under to help maintain proper draping. Before leaving to let him or her get ready, inform the client that you will knock on the door before reentering the room.

- When you return to the room, drape the client's hair just as you would with a facial, with the main objective to protect the hair from any treatments, creams, or muds that will be used. A disposable cap or a hair protector works well for this. This is also a good time to check on your client's comfort level. If necessary, add an additional blanket or fold up the layered ones he or she is lying on, as it is important that the client does not get chilled or overheated during the treatment.

- If the client has chosen not to wear the provided undergarments, properly drape him or her with the modesty towels.

rattling, and running water, to a minimum. Remember, quiet is the key to relaxation.

Proper body temperature and hydration are important too. (See Figures 5–4, 5–5, and 5–6.) Watch for signs of dehydration, especially if your client is using a heated blanket. Always have plenty of drinking water on hand for your clients. You should also monitor your client's body temperature, continually checking to ensure that he or she is never cold. Some clients may be claustrophobic. Your intake forms should include questions to establish what measures are needed to address each client's particular comfort zone.

Ensure your client reaches a full state of relaxation by using the treatment's processing time for hand and foot massages. Add heated mitts or booties. It is also a nice touch to add a scalp massage, when possible. Always look to your client for feedback, letting him know that his comfort is one of your top priorities.

As discussed, modesty is another important aspect of the client's comfort. Many spas provide robes for clients when they are moving from the locker room to their designated treatment room or for use when they are relaxing in a meditation room between treatments. Many of your guests may be spending the whole day at your spa and will find comfort in wearing a robe. When your client is removing or putting on a robe, always step out of the room and knock before reentering.

A clinician can help clients overcome modesty issues by describing the treatment and explaining the draping protocol used during the treatment. For proper draping, use two modesty towels for women and one for men. (See Figure 5–7.) Place a towel over the pelvic area on males and over the pelvic and bust areas for women. Drape the towel and fold back the sheet. Address the area to be treated and then redrape the sheet.

When it is time for the client to roll from a prone or supine position, or vice versa, inform the guest to roll over. Lift the towel or sheet horizontally to your face to ensure the client's privacy. Cover the client with other added blankets or large bath towels. When performing treatments that include the use of foils or plastic after application of treatment products, close and secure the foil or plastic and remove the modesty towels immediately as this makes the client feel more covered.

Help your clients off of the treatment table slowly to avoid injuries, as they may be unsteady from lying down for an extended period of time. During some treatments you may be escorting or helping your client into

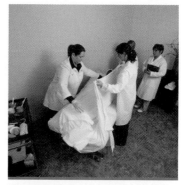

Figure 5–6 Wrapping the client with blankets to further retain heat during the processing portion of the body treatment

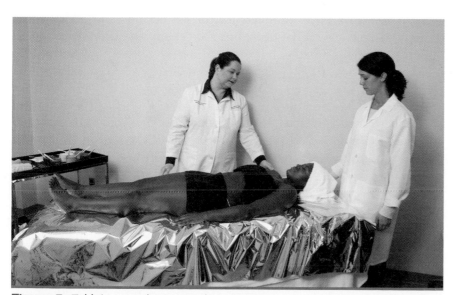

Figure 5–7 Using modesty towels is important for the privacy of the client

the shower. Before helping him or her into the shower, always check the water temperature, setting it to cool, then tepid to help slowly lower the body temperature. If your treatment involves the use of foils or plastic, pull the material up around the legs, back, and chest area for privacy and safety purposes.

Towel Techniques for Product Removal

For those who do not have a wet room available, it can prove messy when trying to remove products such as muds and body masks. One technique that has proven effective is using moist towels heated in a hot towel cabbie. (See Figures 5–8, 5–9, and 5–10.) Begin at the ankle area and place the towel so that it covers the lower portion of the leg. Gently press the towel to the ankle area and begin pushing the towel upward with some pressure to "carry and remove" product from the skin as you work upward to the end of the towel. As you move along, the towel will gather and continue to remove about 99 percent of the product if you are using the proper amount of pressure. Be sure not to press too hard as bony areas could cause discomfort for the client. Once you reach the end, fold the towel in half ensuring that the clean areas of the towel are exposed as the outer portions and use both sides, as necessary to remove any residual product. Place a new towel in the same fashion at the knee, covering up to the upper thigh and use the same press-push-slide technique. Remember to maintain proper draping, exposing only the area you are working on. You may need to practice this, but it is guaranteed to provide great results and easy removal of stubborn products. This technique can be applied to any portion of the body. Some technicians will add moistened and warmed towels over products for further benefits. For added client comfort, dry towels can be heated in the cabbie, and drops of essential oils can also provide further relaxation.

Facial for the Body

When performing a facial for the body, use the same concept and approach that you would for a facial for the face, neck, and décolleté. For this procedure, however, you will cover more area and will need to treat both sides of the body.

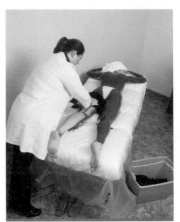

Figure 5–8 Beginning with the legs, push the towel in an upward direction

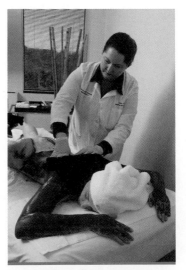

Figure 5–9 If the proper pressure is applied, much of the product can be removed with a towel

■ THE POPULARITY OF BODY WRAPS AND MASKS

Body wraps and masks are growing in popularity, as is demonstrated by the increased number of requests for them in today's spa atmosphere.

One theory for this interest is that the consumer is becoming more educated on the benefits of treating the body as a whole. As a result, many of today's savvy clients are opting for body wraps and masks to combine the relaxation of a massage with the added benefits of a skin treatment. These body treatments range from salt glows and sugar rubs, to full-body herbal wraps and detoxifying paraffin cocoons, to Sedona and French Red Clay Body Masks—all of which work to create truly invigorating spa body treatments for your clients. These treatments are easy to learn as they rely on your fundamental knowledge of performing a facial. (See Table 5–1.)

Common Ingredients Used in Body Treatments

Alpha Hydroxy Acid (AHA): this organic acid taken from fruit acids, is used in antiaging skin care products to encourage moisture restoration, produce exfoliation, and help other ingredients to penetrate through the skin more effectively; must be used in combination with sunscreen

Beta Hydroxy Acid: an oil-soluble organic acid (salicylic acid) used in exfoliators and acne treatments

Caffeine: a stimulant present in coffee, tea, and soda beverages that is also useful to soothe puffy eyes; commonly used in cellulite creams

Camphor: an anti-infective agent with a unique taste and smell that cools and refreshes itchy skin; commonly used to stimulate circulation and refresh the skin in foot treatments

Collagen: the main epidermal protein, is added to topical creams for its moisturizing benefits. (Collagen applied to the skin will not penetrate to produce collagen; it only moisturizes the skin.)

Elastin: a protein in the dermis that is added for its moisturizing effects. (Elastin applied to the skin will not penetrate to produce elastin, it only moisturizes the skin.)

Grape Seed Extract: a botanical extract known to increase the effectiveness of vitamin C by acting as a vehicle and a restorer of oxidized vitamin C

Green Tea Extract: this derivative from decaffeinated green tea contains "catechins," which are effective antioxidants known to help to prevent cancer

Hyaluronic Acid: also known as "cyclic acid," is a powerful moisturizing agent

Hydroquinone: a skin lightening agent

Jojoba Oil: a liquid wax, cold pressed from the seeds of the *Simondsia chinensis;* prized for its humectant and lubricating properties, Jojoba oil closely resembles skin's sebum

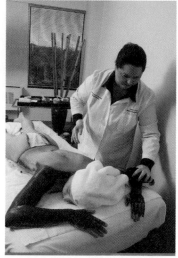

Figure 5–10 Once the towel is full, fold it in half to continue to clean the upper body

Definition of a body wrap:
A body treatment that integrates linens or elastic bandages infused with ingredients to reduce the appearance of cellulite or hydrate the skin.

Definition of a body mask:
A body treatment involving the application of an exfoliating, hydrating, detoxification mask to the entire body.

Table 5–1   Seaweeds and Their Uses

Main Group	General Group Properties	Subgroups	Properties	Recommended Body Condition and Treatment
Algae (alginates)	Aids in skin firmness, cell renewal, and moisturization			
Chlorophyta (green)	Softening, antibacterial, anti-inflammatory	*Lichen moss*		Dry skin, irritation
Cyanophyta (blue-green)	High nutritional group, rich in vitamins A, B, C, E; stimulates cell metabolic rate	*Spirulina*	Rich source of beta-carotene, total food source, sugars (moisturizing), antioxidant	Detox, cellulite, softening, and conditioning
Phaeophyta (brown)	Probably the strongest group for blood and metabolic stimulation	*Laminaria digita*	Sugars (moisturizing), vitamins (antioxidants, etc.); provitamins (carotenoids, vitamin D, etc.); minerals (iodine, etc.); antibacterial, metabolic stimulation	More active treatments using heat and stronger stimulation, detox, cellulite, moisturizing and conditioning, revitalizing
		Fucus Fucus vesibulosus	Similar to *Laminaria digita*	Similar to *Laminaria digita*
Rhodophyta (red)	Contains highly balancing emollient algae	*Chrondrus crispus*	Highly viscous (thick and stabilizing), balancing, emollient (soothing)	Moisturizing and conditioning
		Carageenan	Highly viscous (thick, slippery), emollient (soothing)	Moisturizing and conditioning

Suggested Steps for a Basic Facial for the Body

Prepare the Treatment Room

1. Prepare table with needed materials; outermost layer of material represents the first treatment.

Greet Client

1. Review health history to ensure the treatment(s) to be performed will not be contraindicated with client's health condition.
2. Situate the client on table in prone or supine position according to treatment plan ahead; allow for the least amount of movement by the client.
3. Discuss modesty; keep entire body draped except for part being worked on.

Perform the Body Facial

1. Prepare the body with a cleansing gel or lotion, depending on the client's skin type. Use light effleurage movements over entire body. Rinse with large wet sponges. For a more luxurious feel, use hot moist towels.
2. Spray appropriate toner with the Lucas spray or applicator of your choice. Penetrate the toner until absorption is achieved, using effleurage movements.
3. Apply an exfoliating scrub or granules by hand or with a brush. Massage in a circular motion. For enhanced exfoliation, use a handheld or machine aided brush. For clients with sensitive skin you may omit the exfoliation product and opt for light dry brushing or wet brushing with a cleansing gel or lotion. This is also an appropriate time to use a steamer. For a stand-alone steamer, move it up and down the body, focusing on the area being exfoliated. Rinse with large wet sponges or hot moist towels. Remember to maintain proper draping, exposing only the area you are currently working on.
4. As in Step 2, spray appropriate toner with the Lucas spray or applicator of your choice. Penetrate the toner until absorption is achieved, using light effleurage movements.
5. Apply a massage cream or oil to the body, using light effleurage movements. Rinse off the cream or oil. Spray appropriate toner with the Lucas spray or applicator of your choice. Penetrate the toner until absorption is achieved, using effleurage movements.
6. With a large brush applicator, generously apply the appropriate mask. Allow the mask to process the appropriate length of time. Cover the client well during the mask as he or she may feel cool during the process time. If working on the back of the body, take this time to do a scalp massage. If doing the front of the body, use this time to give the client a hand or foot massage or treatment.
7. Rinse with large wet sponges or hot moist towels.
8. As in Step 2, spray appropriate toner with the Lucas spray or applicator of your choice. Penetrate the toner using effleurage movements until it is absorbed.

Apply a finishing massage cream or oil to the body, using light effleurage movements. At this time you may wish to roll away the sheet the client is lying on to expose a clean surface for him or her to turn over onto. Help the client turn over, maintaining the appropriate draping protocols. Repeat these steps on the other side of the body.

Kaolin: also called China Clay, fine clay that is white in color; kaolin is often used in facial masks and powders that absorb oil

Shea Butter: a fatty butter expressed from the pit of the fruit of the *Butyrosperam parkii* tree; also known as Karite butter; used for its conditioning properties

Sulfur: this essential mineral module of vitamin B that kills bacteria causing acne; found in many masks, especially body treatment products

Vitamin A: a fat-soluble vitamin that keeps skin hydrated; vitamin A is used in skin care products because it improves aging skin and firms skin texture; it can also dry out acne; must be used in conjunction with sunscreens

Vitamin C: a water-soluble vitamin used in cosmetic creams and topical and oral medicines to boost collagen synthesis

Vitamin D: a fat-soluble vitamin; used in some prescription medicines to treat psoriasis

Vitamin E: an oil-soluble antioxidant; used to speed healing and used in products to soften skin

occlusion
accentuates the effects, good or bad, of topical agents

elastic wraps
bandages that can be rolled around a client and have an elastic composition, allowing you to achieve a tight and secure wrap

TYPES OF BODY WRAPS

With all the different types of body treatments that are available today, manufacturers are constantly vying to set their product apart from the competition. Spas are also doing this through the use of ingenious marketing techniques and partnerships with brand names that complement their products and services. Despite all of this effort, most body treatments are similar in technique. It is their ingredients, target, or benefit desired that sets them apart. The clinicians can also distinguish themselves by their touch and how they personalize the treatment.

Body wrap basics involve a wrapping treatment that is applied on top of a mask or treatment. This wrap helps to intensify the treatment by working on the principles of **occlusion**. The wrapping technique prevents the client from becoming cold and allows the product to remain in place.[4] This protocol can be used with most body treatments. The difference would be in the type of wrapping agent or modality used, such as **elastic wraps** or bandages that are wrapped around an individual's legs, arms, and torso, or a full cotton sheet (see Figure 5–11) that wraps the client in a mummy- or cocoon-type position.

The wrapping results in an increase in body temperature, circulation, and dilation of the blood capillaries, which allows the therapeutic ingredients to be absorbed through the pores and hair follicles. The increased body temperature also relaxes tense muscles and increases perspiration

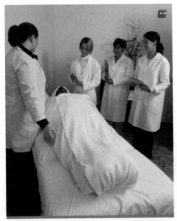

Figure 5–11 A cocoon is the final step in a body wrap treatment

and waste elimination. By adding ingredients such as clays or muds, clients receive the added benefits of drawing out toxins.[5] Elastic wraps are used frequently when clients are trying to receive a temporary slimming effect. The elastic wraps are soaked in a slimming agent or mixture (see Figure 5–12), and pre- and posttreatment measurements are recorded.

Seaweed and Algae Wraps

Seaweed wraps are popular, not only for relaxation purposes, but to stimulate circulation and rid the body of toxins. It is said that seaweed wraps may also address cellulite by providing vitamins and minerals, such as copper, iron, potassium, zinc, and iodine, which can help break up the body's fatty deposits. The overall benefit of seaweed wraps is that the skin looks and feels supple and smooth. The ingredients are composed of micronized algae that can be mixed with warm water. Because the algae have a strong odor, some manufacturers include an additional additive for the client's comfort. You may premix this just prior to your client's arrival and store it in a hot towel cabinet to keep it at a comfortable temperature.

The body is usually exfoliated or dry brushed to stimulate the circulation, and then the algae is applied. (See Figure 5–13.) The treatment begins with an application of a seaweed paste all over the body. Next the area is wrapped with cellophane or warm thermal sheets and processed for approximately 45 minutes. After the seaweed has fully processed, the sheets are removed. The seaweed is rinsed off the body in the shower or removed with warm moist towels.

Advise the client that because the wrap is removing toxins from the skin, it is important to drink extra water for 24 hours before and after the wrap. General contraindications for this treatment include allergies to fish, shellfish, or iodine, which can be major components of the mineralized seaweed powder.

Herbal Wraps

There are several variations on the basic wrapping techniques. These include **herb wraps**, which are herb-soaked linen sheets or elastic wraps resembling ace bandages that are wrapped tightly around the body in a mummy style. The goal of wrapping the client is to create a self-contained system in which the products applied are allowed to interact with the client's body. The beneficial effect of the wrap is achieved by the combination of heat and the properties of the herbs, or from the ingredients applied to the client's skin prior to the wrap.

Each herb has a specific targeted effect. The herbs can assist in increasing the circulation, provide soothing properties and nourishment

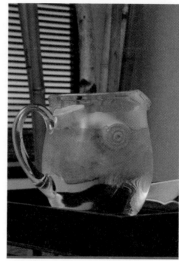

Figure 5–12 Elastic wraps are soaked prior to application

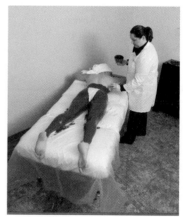

Figure 5–13 The application of a seaweed mask

seaweed wraps
wraps that include application of a seaweed mask followed by a thermal blanket to seal in heat

herb wraps
body wrap treatment that includes the soaking of the wrap in an herbal tea blend prior to applying to the client

Suggested Steps for a Seaweed Wrap

1. Prepare treatment table with protective covering (i.e., sheet, plastic protector sheet, wool blanket, cellophane sheet, or space blanket, and a top sheet or towel). In a bowl, combine the seaweed mixture and prepare for application.

2. Instruct the client to get onto the treatment table just below the top sheet or towel while you step outside the room. Instruct the client to cross the arms (to hold the modesty towel into place) and assist him or her into a sitting up position. Apply the mixture with your hands or an oversized brush to the back and shoulders. Next help the client back to the supine position. Apply the mixture to the legs and buttocks area. Gently raise the knees and apply the mixture to the feet and front and back of the legs, before proceeding to the stomach, chest, and arms. If you prefer, you may first perform any pretreatment exfoliation procedures before applying the seaweed.

3. Begin wrapping the client with plastic wrap and a space blanket while removing the top sheet or towel so that the cellophane is touching the client's skin directly. Next fold up the layers or blankets onto the client. Use a towel around the neck area to prevent heat loss. Process for the desired time, which is usually 25 minutes.

4. Fold down the plastic sheet and blankets. Remove product thoroughly with warm moist towels, redraping as you address each area, or help the client into the shower.

5. Remove all soiled linens so the client will be on a clean dry surface.

6. Apply body lotion or massage cream, using light effleurage movements.

7. Offer the client water for rehydration. Provide information about any specific posttreatment instructions.

diaphoretic
producing or increasing perspiration

hydrocollators
heating units that heat the wrapping linens to an optimal temperature

to the skin, or may be **diaphoretic**. The sheets or bandages are usually soaked in an herbal brew and heated in **hydrocollators**, or heating units, for approximately 20 minutes at 165° Fahrenheit.

The herbs are usually provided in bulk form. Transfer a small amount of these herbal blends to a muslin bag that is filled about three-fourths full. The muslin pouch can be refilled during the day with fresh herbs. You can add more water to the heating unit. It is recommended to start each day with a new batch or, if not, that a fresh brew is made every other day. The mixture may be stored overnight in the refrigerator. It is a good idea to have several bags of the herbs available for your clients to purchase for home use.

When retrieving the linens or wraps, protect your hands from the heat by using rubber gloves. Simple wood clamps can help when wringing the heavy muslin sheets out of the heating units and steaming herbal solution.

Once the herbal wrap is applied, the person is then covered with a blanket, and a cold compress is applied to the forehead. The treatment typically processes for approximately 30 minutes. Some spas use infrared heating lamps to keep clients warm. Remember that an herbal wrap is a heated treatment. As such, it is contraindicated for anyone who has open wounds or sores, is pregnant, has hypertension, as well as for those suffering from circulatory disorders, heart conditions, decreased feelings of sensation, or diabetes. This treatment may also not be appropriate for clients who tend to feel claustrophobic.[6]

Popular Herbals

Today many clients are asking for all natural or herbal body baths, treatments, and facials. (See Table 5–2.) As an aesthetician, it is important to understand the basics of them and to have a few natural therapies on your menu of services. Before doing so, be sure to familiarize yourself with the lists of herbs and essential oils and what they do.

Understanding herbs does not require a scientific degree. Take, for example, the use of the herb **patchouli**. It is fresh or dried leaves mixed with essential oils, and it is used for several therapeutic purposes. It is well

patchouli
an essential oil derived from the leaves of the patchouli scrub

Table 5–2	Ingredients for an Herbal Scrub	
Ingredients	**Benefit and Function**
Liquid soap base	Cleansing
Finely ground oat powder	Soothing
Honey	Moisturizing; antibacterial
Almond meal	Moisturizing
Walnut leaf powder	Skin cell regeneration; weakened cell reconstitution
Apricot kernel oil	Nutritious
Vitamin E oil	Antioxidant

Preparation for an Herbal Body Wrap Treatment

Fill the heating unit nearly three quarters full with water to allow for submersion of herbs and wrap sheets. After the water reaches 165° Fahrenheit, completely submerge a herb-filled muslin pouch in it. Allow the herbal mix to brew for approximately 20 to 30 minutes. After the herbs have completely brewed, you will have an herbal tea. Submerse two wrap sheets in the tea, allowing them to soak for 20 minutes. While the sheets are soaking, prepare the treatment table with a wool or thick blanket followed by a thermal blanket or plastic sheet to protect any underlying linens or blankets.

To ensure your client receives the full benefits of this treatment, instruct him to avoid showering immediately after the wrap as the herbs continue to work for several hours. Also stress the importance of rest and replenishing any water loss that has occurred during this treatment. Remind the client to drink plenty of water to continue the detoxification process.

Suggested Steps for an Herbal Body Wrap

1. Begin the treatment with a light massage, using effleurage movements or by dry brushing the area to be treated. Dry brushing helps remove dead skin cells and stimulates the lymphatic system.
2. Remove one of the soaked linen sheets (wear proper hand protection to avoid burns) and place it on the bed, creating a long rectangle, which allows the sides to be folded up around the client. Lay client inside the sheet, wrapping linen quickly around the entire body. Remove the second linen, and place it on top of the client so that the sheet is doubled to allow more heat conservation.
3. Wrap the thermal blanket over the herbal wrap sheet.
4. Wrap the wool blanket over the thermal blanket. Use a towel around the neck area to prevent heat loss. A second wool blanket can be placed on top for additional heat retention.
5. Apply a cool, folded washcloth to the client's forehead. For additional comfort a pillow may also be placed under the head and bolstered under knees.
6. Leave the client wrapped for 20 to 30 minutes. At this time, do a scalp massage or allow the client to relax to soothing music.

After the wrap has processed, remove the layers. Allow the client to become acclimated before assisting him or her off of the table.

regarded for its positive effect on skin infections, eczema, acne, and chapped skin, as well as for the promotion of cell rejuvenation and the tightening of loose skin. Other uses of its essential oils include antidepressant effects, antiseptic, astringent, deodorant, diuretic, fungicide, insecticide, and sedative properties.[7]

Sometimes the oil extracted from a particular plant is what you will use during treatments; other times it will be some form of the herb itself. (See Figure 5–14.) The herbal form, though not as strong as the essential oil, still poses a health risk to some clients. Because of this, the use of herbs and essential oils require extensive training. Before using any of them, you need to be aware of the many contraindications associated with them.

One of the common uses for herbs is the herbal bath. Herbal baths and medicinal bathing (also referred to as **thalassotherapy** or hydrotherapy) was traditionally utilized as a cosmetic, hygienic, and medicinal treatment. Herbal baths were employed in the treatment of skin conditions, including acne, dermatitis, eczema, psoriasis, and scalp itching, flaking, and dandruff. Herbal bath teas combine benefits of herbal aromatherapy and direct application of herbal nutrients to the skin. They are used as a body bath, a footbath, an herbal wrap, and an aromatherapy herbal pillow.[8]

Herbal scrubs are fairly easy to perform, and the results are easily repeatable. Start off with your soap base and mix ingredients into the soap, one at a time until you have achieved a paste. Massage into the skin, working up a creamy lather. Rinse off, using a warm moist towel to

thalassotherapy
the therapeutic use of the beneficial effects of sea water

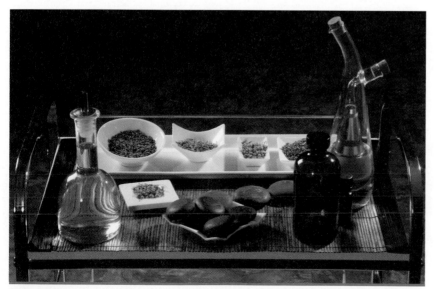

Figure 5–14 Herbs and other items used in body wraps and body treatments

Table 5–3   Herbs Used in Wraps[9]

Herb	Form	Benefit
Allspice	Berry	Effective with arthritis and sore muscles; mild anesthetic
Basil	Leaf	Stimulating
Burdock	Root	Relieves bruises and inflammation
Clove	Stems	Astringent properties
Comfrey	Leaf	Soothing
Eucalyptus	Leaf	Increases blood circulation
Ginger	Root	Increases circulation; detoxifying agent
Lavender	Flower	Soothing
Rosemary	Leaf	Astringent; toning; stimulating
Sage	Leaf	Muscle relaxant

Be aware of any contraindications and your client's health history before integrating the use of herbs into your therapies. For example, rosemary is contraindicative to individuals with high blood pressure, and clove and allspice can be very skin sensitizing, so use sparingly.

aromatherapy
the use of essential oils in lotions and inhalants in an effort to affect mood and promote health

remove. Add a light moisturizer, if needed, or proceed with your next treatment.[10]

The herbs found in an herbal wrap typically consist of detoxifying, toning, stimulating, or relaxing and soothing herbs. (See Table 5–3.) Detoxifying herbs may include eucalyptus, clove, rosemary, and ginger root. Soothing and relaxing herbs may include bergamot, cedar, chamomile, jasmine, patchouli, marjoram, sage, lavender, comfrey, and burdock. Each body wrap will differ from manufacturer to manufacturer, as well as according to its target and action desired.[11]

Essential Oil Wrap

Aromatherapy is the therapeutic use of plant aromas for beauty and health treatment purposes. Aromatherapy in the context of spa treatments is the use of essential oils during facials, massages, and body treatments. These services incorporate essential oils at different times during the treatment for various therapeutic benefits.

The most common method involves applying the essential oils by massaging the diluted oils onto the body. The essential oil is always mixed with carrier oil and is never applied directly to the body. Application of diluted oils should be done after the wrap due to the fact that this could increase sensitivity or the client could have a toxic overload. Another effective use would be adding a scent to your linens or towels,

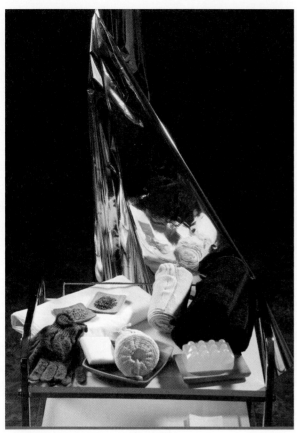

Figure 5–15 Wrap materials can vary and include Mylar and blankets

dispersing the aroma into the air during the treatments or by performing a scalp massage with aromatic oils. Because learning about essential oils, proper mixing protocols, their indications, and contraindications requires extensive education, manufacturers have taken the guesswork out by providing kits and ready-to-use treatments. It is advisable that you take advantage of these resources rather than putting your client at risk. When using essential oils, be very aware of the contraindications and your client's health history.[12] (See Figure 5–15 and Table 5–4.)

Cellophane, Space Blankets, or Foil Wrapping Agents

A foil or **cellophane body wrap** is designed to aid in the detoxification process by locking in heat, moisture, vitamins, and minerals. It is

cellophane body wrap
a wrap that uses a plastic material to aid in the penetration of the product through the principal of occlusion

Table 5–4 Supplies Needed for Wrap and Masks[13]	
Treatment table	According to service
Disposable undergarments	For client (or use modesty towels)
Treatment gown	For client modesty, depending on treatment
Headband or hair wrap	To protect the hair
Clean bandages, plastic, cellophane, metallic spa sheet, or space blanket	Clean bandages, plastic, metallic spa sheet (depends on treatment)
Tape measure	To measure the client before and after treatment if performing a slimming body wrap
Bowls	To mix products as needed
Spatulas/brushes	To apply treatment products
Water	Used to mix with powder ingredients and masks. It is also advised to have a glass of water for the client to drink readily available.
Treatment products	Clays, masks, herbs, essential oils, marine algae, or seaweed
Thermal blankets	To maintain heat (if required)
Client record card	To assess client and record details of treatment
Shower facility	To cleanse the skin before treatment and remove treatment products following a treatment
Hot, steamed towels	To remove product if the workplace does not have a shower facility

designed to work with the body's own natural heat. The benefit of using these items is that in most cases they are disposable. Once you begin to work with algae, seaweeds, and some masks, you will realize they stain the linens. Foil or cellophane wrap agents can form a protective barrier between the solutions used in your treatment and your linens. (See Figure 5–16.)

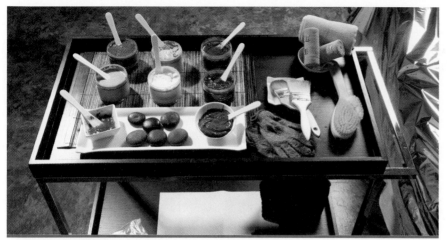

Figure 5–16 The inventory of supplies for body wraps and masks can be extensive

▪ BLANKET WRAPS

Blanket wraps are used in place of the elastic body wrap. The application of a blanket after a treatment is used to maintain heat or to cool the body. A typical blanket wrap procedure may include a mud bath followed by a shower, a soak in a mineral bath, or relaxation time in a steam room. This is followed by a wrap with a large cotton blanket that envelops the client like a cocoon for quiet and relaxation. The blanket wrap may be followed with a massage. This series truly demonstrates a full body spa experience.[14] (See Figure 5–17.)

Dry Blanket Wraps or Cool Moist Blanket Wraps

A dry blanket wrap can be used after the client's core body temperature has increased in heated water or body treatment. It begins with a first layer wrapping in a light cotton blanket, then with a heavier wool one. This accelerates the release of toxins from the body. It is always recommended that the client drink plenty of water afterwards to help rehydrate his or her system.

In the instances of cool moist blanket wraps, the goal is to cool the client. In the case of treating sensitized or sunburned skin, an aloe vera mixture may be applied to the first blanket the client is wrapped in and then followed by another, to prevent evaporation. Cool moist

blanket wraps
the application of a blanket after a treatment to maintain heat or to cool the body

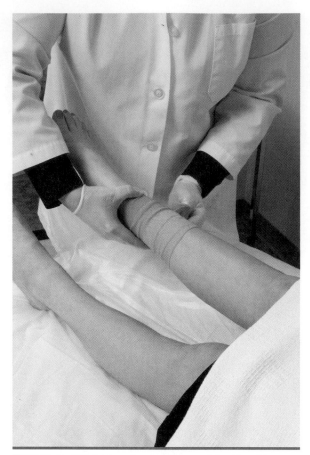

Figure 5–17 Leg wraps are used for tired legs

blanket wraps can also be used to promote a soothing and comforting outcome.[15]

Kneipp Body Wraps

Kneipp Body Wraps
envelops a body part with wet and dry cloths that are either hot or cold; effects are achieved through temperature, length of application, and additives

The **Kneipp Body Wraps** were developed by Bavarian monk, Father Sebastian Kneipp, who believed that disease could be cured by using water to eliminate waste from the body and that the cornerstone of health was through life-style, health education, and self-responsibility. Kneipp developed over 100 different hydrotherapy treatments using water in solid, liquid, and vapor forms. His treatments included washings, wraps, packs, compresses, steam, and baths.

A Kneipp wrap envelops a body part with wet and dry cloths that are either hot or cold. Effects are achieved through temperature, length of application, and additives. Increased circulation promotes the removal

Suggested Steps for a Soothing Leg Treatment

You will need a bottle of Italian mineral water, bottled at the source of a hot or thermal spring. The water will be used in place of toner and used to rinse the skin instead of regular water. This will help remineralize the skin and prevent stripping of the acid mantle usually caused by chlorine and processing by-products in normal tap water. You will also need cotton bandages or cloths to wrap the legs in.

1. Prepare the treatment table with protective covering (i.e., sheet, plastic protector sheet, and a top sheet or towel). Place a mixture of thermal or mineral water, fango mud, and exfoliating granules in a bowl and prepare for application.
2. Instruct the client to get onto the treatment table just below the top sheet or towel while you step outside the room.
3. On moistened skin, begin application of a mixture of thermal or mineral water, fango mud, and exfoliating granules and apply at the feet and work up the legs in an upward and gentle circular motion using the hands. Be careful to avoid any scratched or wounded areas. (Remember to consider the client's skin type when choosing the level of exfoliation.)
4. Gently raise the knees. Apply the mixture to the feet and front and back of the legs. Pay special attention to dryer areas, such as the heels of the feet and the elbows, if necessary.
5. Using the same steps as above, remove the product thoroughly with warm, moist towels (redraping as each area is addressed) or assist the client into the shower. If your client is not showering, roll or fold away the plastic protector sheet to provide a clean surface for him or her to lie on. It is important to remove all traces of the exfoliating mud because it will not prove relaxing when applying any afterproducts or continuing with other treatments. (You may rinse with warmed towels moistened with thermal or mineral water and heated in the hot towel cabbie.)
6. Choose a mineralizing cream or nourishing cream and mix together with an ampoule that is mineralizing or stress relieving. Apply mixture of ampoule and cream. Layer fango mud and leave in place for 20 minutes, covering the area with a thermal or heated blanket.
7. Soak cotton cloths in cooled thermal or mineral water and place (wrap) around lower legs. Allow client to rest.

Choose a stimulating or camphor based cream, mineralizing cream, or nourishing cream and complete the treatment with a stimulating, drainage massage or use a pressotherapy treatment machine.

of metabolic wastes and increases the oxygen and nutrient supply to the skin, resulting in a healthy glow.[16]

History and Use of the Vichy Shower

The vichy shower is thought to have originated in Vichy, France. Vichy's hot mineral springs have made it one of the foremost spas in Europe. The first step to beginning a shower treatment is to empty the water pipes of the water that has been standing and has become cold and to adjust the water temperature. The client must not be under the showerhead when it is first turned on or during the temperature adjustment phase. The temperature must not exceed 104° Fahrenheit. Once the optimal temperature has been achieved, you will close the valve briefly while the client is positioned onto the table. Once the client is comfortable, you will open the valve and adjust the angle and volume of the heads as desired. The second step is to adjust the intensity to the desired pressure. The pressures range from a fine mist to a jet stream and can be adjusted by twisting the head valves. It is best to drain all water from the heads between treatments by opening and closing the showerhead valves until the water is absent.

A **Scotch hose** is a hose that projects water through a jet hose that stimulates the client from 10 to 12 feet away. Therapists are expertly trained to massage the client in specific patterns. When operating the Scotch hose you must remember to always hold the hose when turning on the water and never let go of the nozzle when the water is flowing. You will remove the hose from the nozzle holder, turn on the water, and initially direct it toward the floor and drain until you have achieved an optimal temperature never exceeding 104° Fahrenheit. When increasing or decreasing the pressure, please note that this too will affect the temperature. After using the hose to deliver an invigorating massage, empty the water from the hose and return the hose to the nozzle holder.[17]

Scotch hose
a hose similar to a fire hose used in water therapy

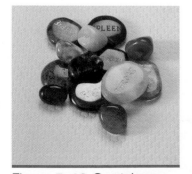

Figure 5–18 Crystals are used on the chakra points during massage or a facial

Enhancing Massage with Crystals

Although scientific studies have not yet been conducted on crystals and gemstones, crystals and color therapy have been used for centuries to energetically alter the body and treat illness. The use of crystals in the spa has gained popularity. You may use crystals on the chakra points during massage or a facial. Crystals and cold stones may also be used during the masking portion of a facial on the eyes to reduce inflammation and soreness.[18] (See Figure 5–18.)

Conclusion

When working in a spa there are many items to consider, not just the services you offer clients. Confidentiality, privacy, health screening, indications and contraindications, and client preparation and comfort are all important factors to consider. There are an unlimited number of spa body treatments available to you today to offer to your clients. First consider the space and equipment available. You should also investigate your market and decide which treatments best fit your clientele. Today's full service spa offers a wide array of body treatments and hydrotherapy services including body wraps and masks, vichy showers, and hydrotherapy tubs.

▶ ⟩ ⟩ TOP 10 TIPS TO TAKE TO THE CLINIC

1. Choose the best treatment table you can afford.
2. Protect your clients' files in a locked cabinet.
3. Let your clients know your policies on privacy.
4. Choose a few treatments to focus on.
5. Offer monthly promotions to spotlight different treatments.
6. Prepare your treatments well ahead of time.
7. Design take-home informational sheets to help your clients maintain results at home.
8. Always do a heath screening to prevent contraindications to treatments.
9. Have water available for clients to drink to prevent dehydration.
10. Never leave a client unattended during a treatment.

CHAPTER QUESTIONS

1. What steps are important in preparing a client?
2. Why is client comfort important?
3. Why should you choose a reliable table?
4. Why should you protect the client's privacy?
5. Name several types of body treatments.
6. Which treatments require a shower?

7. What are blanket wraps?

8. What is a vichy shower?

CHAPTER REFERENCES

1. D'Angelo, J., Dean, P., Deitz, S., Hinds, C., Lees, M., Miller, E., et al. (2003). *Milady's Standard: Comprehensive Training for Estheticians.* Clifton Park, NY: Thomson Delmar Learning.

2. D'Angelo, J., Dean, P., Deitz, S., Hinds, C., Lees, M., Miller, E., et al. (2003). *Milady's Standard: Comprehensive Training for Estheticians.* Clifton Park, NY: Thomson Delmar Learning.

3. Decrko, J. P., Domar, A. D., & Deckro, R. M. (1999). Clinical Application of the Relaxation Response in Women's Health. *AWHONN's Clinical Issues in Perinatal and Women's Health Nursing, 4*(2), 311–319.

4. Worwood, V. (2001). *Aromatherapy for the Beauty Therapist.* Clifton Park, NY: Thomson Delmar Learning.

5. Nordmann, L. (2002). *Professional Beauty Therapy, The Official Guide to Level 3.* Clifton Park, NY: Thomson Delmar Learning.

6. Worwood, V. (2001). *Aromatherapy for the Beauty Therapist.* Clifton Park, NY: Thomson Delmar Learning.

7. Decrko, J. P., Domar, A. D., & Deckro, R. M. (1999). Clinical Application of the Relaxation Response in Women's Health. *AWHONN's Clinical Issues in Perinatal and Women's Health Nursing, 4*(2), 311–319.

8. Worwood, V. (2001). *Aromatherapy for the Beauty Therapist.* Clifton Park, NY: Thomson Delmar Learning.

9. Worwood, V. (2001). *Aromatherapy for the Beauty Therapist.* Clifton Park, NY: Thomson Delmar Learning.

10. Worwood, V. (2001). *Aromatherapy for the Beauty Therapist.* Clifton Park, NY: Thomson Delmar Learning.

11. Worwood, V. (2001). *Aromatherapy for the Beauty Therapist.* Clifton Park, NY: Thomson Delmar Learning.

12. Worwood, V. (2001). *Aromatherapy for the Beauty Therapist.* Clifton Park, NY: Thomson Delmar Learning.

13. Worwood, V. (2001). *Aromatherapy for the Beauty Therapist.* Clifton Park, NY: Thomson Delmar Learning.

14. Nordmann, L. (2002). *Professional Beauty Therapy, The Official Guide to Level 3.* Clifton Park, NY: Thomson Delmar Learning.

15. Bergel, R., & Leavy, H. (2003). *The Spa Encyclopedia.* Clifton Park, NY: Thomson Delmar Learning.

16. Bergel, R., & Leavy, H. (2003). *The Spa Encyclopedia*. Clifton Park, NY: Thomson Delmar Learning.
17. Bergel, R., & Leavy, H. (2003). *The Spa Encyclopedia*. Clifton Park, NY: Thomson Delmar Learning.
18. http://altmedicine.about.com

Lymphatic Drainage and Cellulite Treatments

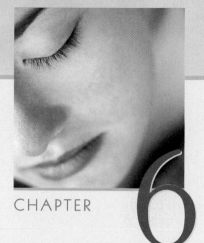

CHAPTER 6

KEY TERMS

adaptive immunity

cellulite

edema

initial lymphatics

innate immunity

obstructive lymphedema

primary lymphoid organs

secondary lymphoid organs

stationary circle

thoracic duct

watersheds

LEARNING OBJECTIVES

After completing this chapter, you should be able to:

1. Discuss the benefits of lymphatic drainage.
2. Discuss the indications and contraindications of lymphatic drainage.
3. Discuss the immune system and components.
4. Discuss edema and its causes.
5. Discuss cellulite and its causes.
6. Discuss suggested treatments for lymphatic drainage and cellulite.

▪ THE HISTORY OF LYMPHATIC DRAINAGE

I n Europe the average aesthetician spends two years in aesthetician college and learns to be proficient in both face and body protocols. Aestheticians in Europe use *lymphatic drainage* in most of their face and body treatments because they fully grasp the benefits this modality offers. American trained aestheticians are just beginning to understand the implications of its use and are beginning to implement it as an integral part of face and body treatments.

Emil and Estrid Vodder, Danish physical therapists, developed the Vodder Manual Lymph Drainage techniques in the 1930s. Lymph drainage is also known as lymphatic drainage or lymphatic drainage massage. The Vodder method involves light, rhythmic manipulations in order to stimulate lymph flow and fluid movement. Until the recent increase in the popularity of lymphatic drainage and in the wealth of information available, the Vodder method was one of only a few methods of lymphatic drainage available. Since its development in the 1930s, there have been leaps and bounds in research focused on lymphatic drainage and its techniques. More scientific studies have been conducted; research and advances in technology have given rise to more effective techniques of lymphatic drainage than the original version of the earlier methods. With the more modernized methods of lymphatic drainage, aestheticians can easily integrate lymphatic drainage into their esthetic protocols and achieve even greater effects than Emil and Estrid Vodder ever dreamed of.

Ponce de Leon was always searching for the fountain of youth, but it may be closer than he thought. Research has demonstrated that lymphatic drainage accelerates the flow of lymphatic fluid in the lymph ducts to the lymph nodes where toxins are filtered and eliminated. As a result, the skin is better able to purge the toxins that build up from chemicals in our food and our environment, as well as wastes that are a result of normal cellular metabolism.

Lymphatic drainage should be considered as a valuable tool for the aesthetician. Modern techniques use gentle, external massage strokes with precise rhythm, pressure, and speed to mimic the action of the lymphatic system in a specific sequence, according to the desired effect. (See Figure 6–1.) It is beneficial for increasing the healing process, effective for use in pre- and post-op treatments, and beneficial for all skin types. It is great for acne clients, as well as effective for detoxification, edema, cellulite, and sluggish complexions. Lymphatic drainage can easily be consid-

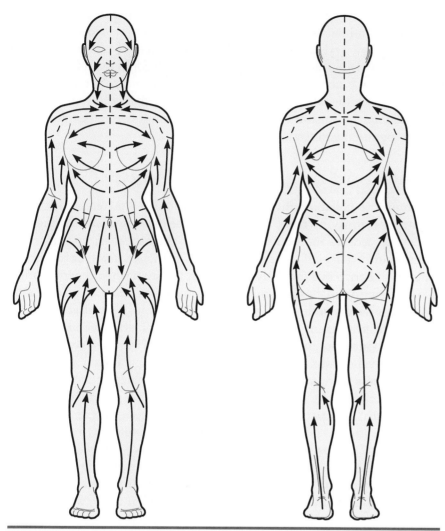

Figure 6–1 Lymph drainage massage encourages lymph fluid to follow its natural path

ered a full cleansing experience for all the layers of the skin and the body as a whole. The result is whole body, a more clarified and clear complexion, reduction in puffiness and dark circles in the eye area, reduction in whole body or site specific edema, and even reduction in fine line wrinkles.

The Immune System

To fully comprehend the effectiveness of the use of lymph drainage in aesthetics treatments, it is important to understand some of the structure and function of the *immune system*.

The immune system evolved to protect multicellular organisms from pathogens. Pathogens are grouped into four major categories: viruses, bacteria, fungi, and parasites. The immune system is highly adaptable to effectively defend against foreign invaders. All components act together as a dynamic network. It is very complex and includes an enormous variety of molecules and cells that are capable of recognizing and targeting foreign invaders. In short, the immune system has two important activities, recognition and response.

Innate and Adaptive Immunity

innate immunity
the resistance to disease that a species possesses at birth

adaptive immunity
antigen-specific immune response as a result of exposure to the specific antigen; for example, chicken pox

There are two collaborating systems of immunity, innate and adaptive. **Innate immunity** involves molecular and cellular mechanisms that are already present as the body's first line of defense when encountering infection or invaders. The first hurdle for a pathogen involves breeching anatomical barriers of the body. Acidity in the stomach and perspiration are protective against organisms that are unable to survive in acidic environments. Tears contain enzymes called lysozymes that attack the cell walls of the invader on contact. The skin is also an effective barrier, and this is why burn victims usually have to be treated aggressively with preventative medications to fight off bacterial and fungal infections. Beyond initial barriers there are pattern recognition molecules and other highly effective components. Present are cells such as phagocytes that work to ingest extracellular particulate material (phagocytosis) and antimicrobial compounds such as interferons (proteins that bind to cells to produce an antiviral state), lysozymes (enzymes that break down cell walls of invaders), and collectins (proteins that kill bacteria by disrupting lipid membranes). All work by the ability to recognize and neutralize invaders.

The second form of immunity is **adaptive immunity**, which develops as a response to an invader, retaining the memory and in the future being able to recognize and then eliminate it. Innate and adaptive immunities work in tangent as a highly cooperative system. Innate immunity works within hours, has a limited and fixed specificity, and recognizes only a limited number of invaders, whereas adaptive immunity has a response time of days and the specificity is highly diverse and actually improves during the course of the immune response. Major components of adaptive immunity include lymphocytes, antigen specific receptors, and antibodies. Antigens include foreign proteins, viruses, bacteria, fungi, and parasites. In studies it has been found that both lymphocytes and antigen-presenting cells cooperate during the process of adaptive immunity. There are two types of lymphocytes: B lymphocytes (B cells) and T lymphocytes (T cells). B lymphocytes are mature in bone marrow and express unique antigen binding receptors on its membrane.

After an initial encounter with an antigen, the B cells differentiate into antibody secreting plasma cells, and the antibody binds with the antigen and facilitates the invaders' clearance from the body. T lymphocytes are also found in bone marrow but migrate to the thalamus to mature and express a unique antigen binding receptor on its membrane. T cells recognize antigens that are directly bound to their membranes, not free-floating antigens as with the B cells. Once the antigen is bound (now called altered self-cell), the T cells recognize the antigen and respond by producing cytokines. Cytotoxic T lymphocytes (CTLs) mediate the killing of the (bound) altered self-cells.

On occasion the immune system does function improperly. This can mean it fails to protect the host properly or, in some instances, it can overreact in the cases of allergies, asthma, autoimmune disease, or immunodeficiency.

Cells and Organs of the Immune System

There are two main groups of cells, organs, and tissues of the immune system, primary lymphoid organs and secondary lymphoid organs. **Primary lymphoid organs** are responsible for providing an environment conducive for the development and maturation of lymphocytes. **Secondary lymphoid organs** are responsible for trapping antigens and are sites where mature lymphocytes can eliminate the antigens.

The lymph organs, blood, and lymphatic fluid contain white blood cells (leukocytes). Normal adult blood contains red blood cells, platelets, and leukocytes. The leukocyte category includes cells that help participate in the immune response called lymphocytes, granulocytes, platelets, monocytes, and macrophages. Lymphoid cells include B cells, T cells, and natural killer (NK) cells. NK cells do not synthesize antigen specific receptors; most display only a T cell receptor that recognizes and binds specific antigens. NK cells display cytotoxic activity against tumors and cells infected with some viruses and are part of the innate immune system. Granulocytes are classified as neutrophils, eosinophils, and basophiles. There are mast cells, dendritic cells, and follicular dendritic cells (located in the structures of the lymph node called lymph follicles) as well. Macrophages and neutrophils (the first to arrive at the site of inflammation) are specialized cells capable of phagocytosis of antigens. Eosinophils are motile phagocytic cells and can move from blood to tissue with ease. Basophiles are responsible for releasing chemicals that lead to allergic responses. Dendritic cells (DCs), identified by Paul Langerhans in 1868, capture antigens to present to T cells. There are four categories of dendritic cells: Langerhans DCs (located in the epidermis), interstitial DCs (located in all interstitial spaces of organs except the brain),

primary lymphoid organs
thymus and bone marrow

secondary lymphoid organs
lymph nodes, tonsils, lymph follicles of the mucous membranes, and the white pulp of the spleen

monocyte-derived DCs (arise from monocytes that have migrated into tissues) and plasmacytoid-derived DCs (arise from plasmacytoid cells and act as antigen presenting cells). All four are derived from hematopoietic stem cells.

Organs of the Immune System

The organs of the immune system can be grouped onto two sections and can be distinguished by function: the primary lymphoid organs and secondary lymphoid organs.

Primary lymph organs are the sites where lymphocytes develop, and secondary lymphoid organs are where the lymphocytes encounter the antigen. Primary lymphoid organs in mammals include bone marrow and thymus. Secondary lymphoid organs in mammals include lymph nodes, spleen, and mucosal-associated lymphoid tissue. (See Figure 6–2.) When foreign invaders enter the tissues, they are picked up by the lymphatic system and are carried into various lymph tissues and the lymph nodes.

Primary Lymphoid Organs

All cells of the blood originate from pluripotent stem cells in the bone marrow. Animals, including humans, will die when given high dose radiation because stem cells will be destroyed. Bone marrow also serves as the site of maturation of B lymphocytes.

The thymus is an organ situated above the heart and below the thyroid gland. Each lobe is surrounded by a capsule and is divided into lobules, which are separated from each other by strands of connective tissue called trabeculae. Each lobule is organized into two compartments: the cortex (outer compartment) and the medulla (inner compartment).

The thymus is at its largest relative size at birth and its largest actual size is at puberty. Following puberty the thymus begins to shrink so that in elderly individuals hardly any of it is left. There is a relationship between aging and a decline in immune responsiveness. Stress can also result in shrinkage of the thymus.

Secondary Lymphoid Organs

Lymph nodes serve as the first organized structures to encounter most antigens. Lymph nodes are encapsulated bean-shaped structures containing a reticular network packed with lymphocytes, macrophages, and dendritic cells. They are present at the junctions of lymphatic vessels. The

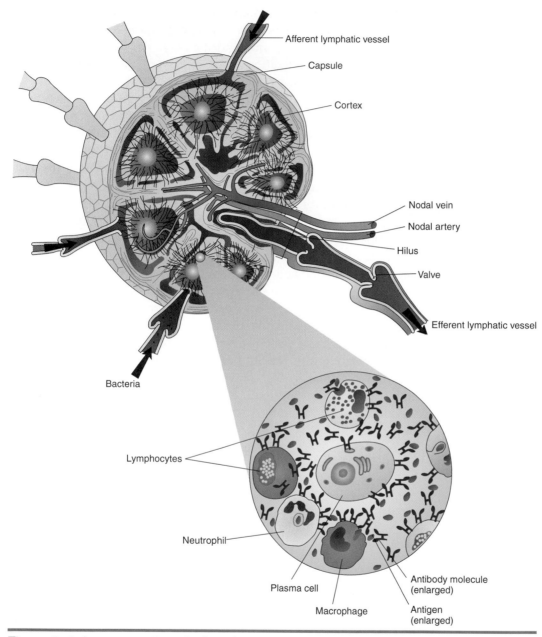

Afferent lymphatic vessel

Capsule

Cortex

Nodal vein

Nodal artery

Hilus

Valve

Efferent lymphatic vessel

Bacteria

Lymphocytes

Neutrophil

Plasma cell

Macrophage

Antibody molecule
(enlarged)

Antigen
(enlarged)

Figure 6–2 A cross-section of a lymph node

major function of the lymph nodes is to filter antigen from the lymph. The lymph node contains three regions. The cortex is the outermost layer and contains mostly B lymphocytes, follicular dendritic cells, and macrophages arranged in clusters called primary follicles. Following antigenic stimulation, the primary follicles become secondary follicles consisting of concentric rings of densely packed lymphocytes and central lymphocytes, macrophages, and dendritic cells. The GCs (germinal centers) contain large proliferating B lymphocytes and plasma cells interspersed with macrophages and dendritic cells. The GC is a site of intense B cell activation and differentiation into plasma cells and memory cells. The paracortex is the layer just beneath the cortex and is populated with T lymphocytes and dendritic cells. This layer is an important site for T cell activation. The medulla is the innermost layer, contains fewer cell populations, and consists mostly of plasma cells. Afferent lymphatic vessels pierce the capsule of a *lymph node* (vessels leading into the node) at various sites and empty into the subcapsular sinus. There is a single efferent lymphatic vessel leading from the lymph node with high antibody concentrations. An afferent artery enters the lymph node and is where lymphocytes pass in between specialized capillary endothelial cells in the postcapillary venules. Swollen lymph nodes can be attributed to the concentration of lymphocytes in the lymph nodes.

Lymph is fluid from the tissues that flows from the intercellular tissue spaces into lymphatic capillaries and then into a series of larger collecting vessels called lymphatic vessels. *Lymphatic vessels* converge into the thoracic duct, which returns the fluid to the circulatory system by dumping into the left subclavian vein. The **initial lymphatics** carry the lymph through lymph nodes, where it filters through a cellular network containing reticular dendritic cells and phagocytic cells that trap antigens carried by the lymph.

The spleen is a large, oval secondary lymphoid organ positioned high in the left abdominal cavity. The spleen is adapted to filter the blood; it responds, therefore, to systemic infections. The spleen is not supplied by afferent lymphatics. Bloodborne cells and antigens are carried into the spleen through the splenic artery, which empties into the marginal zone. Antigen enters the marginal zone, and it is trapped by interdigitating dendritic cells, which carry the antigen to the periarteriolar lymphoid sheath (PALS). More recirculating lymphocytes pass daily through the spleen than all of the lymph nodes combined. A variety of other lymphoid tissues are found at various locations along mucous membrane surfaces (digestive system, respiratory system, and urogenital system); these tissues are called mucosal-associated lymphoid tissue (MALT). MALT appears to be secondary lymphoid tissue. There are organized clusters of MALT: tonsils, appendix, and Peyer's patches. The tonsils are grouped into three locations: lingual at the base of the tongue, palatine at the side of the back of the mouth, and nasopharyngeal in the roof of the nasopharynx (adenoids).

initial lymphatics
interstitial fluid that first enters the lymph system and becomes lymph fluid

Functions of the Lymphatic System

Functions of the lymphatic system include balancing fluid, distributing immune cells to maintain health, ridding tissues of excess protein, carrying digested fat to blood vessels, repairing injured tissues, and regenerating new lymph nodes in infected areas.

Proteins that are left in tissue can cause an inflammatory response that includes pain, swelling, and scar tissue buildup, and can also be life threatening. The openings to blood vessels are too small to absorb the proteins as well as other molecules. It is therefore the responsibility of the lymph system to absorb the proteins and release them back into the bloodstream.

When tissue is injured, chemicals from the damaged cells cause inflammation. Blood circulation increases and fluid is released to the damaged area. Immune cells wall off the injured area and destroy harmful organisms. The lymph system transports immune cells throughout the body. Immune cells create antibodies for every disease-causing microorganism they encounter, which then destroys it.

Lymph Fluid Flow

Lymph is body fluid consisting of water, electrolytes, and proteins. It is initiated when blood pressure forces plasma to seep out of blood capillaries into tissue spaces. An average adult will produce 2.9 liters or more during a 24-hour period. When in the interstitial space, it is considered interstitial fluid; it bathes, nourishes tissue cells, and picks up foreign particles, enzymes, and proteins. When this fluid does not return to circulation, edema will result. **Edema** is a progressive swelling and can eventually become life threatening. Under normal conditions, some of the interstitial fluid is returned to the blood via capillary walls while the remainder of the interstitial fluid is absorbed into the tiny networks of lymphatic capillaries consisting of a loose network of endothelial cells. Lymph capillaries contain one way valves that allow fluid to enter. These openings are variable and can widen when there is more fluid in the tissues but have no smooth muscle cells like blood capillaries. The *bicuspid valves* prevent backward movement of the lymph when the vessel compresses. The vessel can contract from increased tissue pressure. At this time, the valve that the fluid entered from closes up and the valve connecting to the next lymphangion opens up. The process continues on in a wavelike contraction. Lymph then flows from the tiny network of vessels to the larger collection vessels called lymphatic vessels. The largest lymphatic vessel, the **thoracic duct** empties into the left subclavian

edema
swelling resulting from excessive fluid buildup in tissue

thoracic duct
the main duct of the lymphatic system, ascending through the thoracic cavity in front of the spinal column

vein and receives lymph fluid from all parts of the body except the right arm and the right side of the body. The right lymphatic duct collects lymph from the upper right side of the body and the right arm and drains into the right subclavian vein. The lymph fluid is then recycled into the blood.

The three main factors that assist in lymph circulation are muscular contraction, movement, and pressure changes. The two stages of lymph circulation are the absorption of lymph into the initial lymphatics and the propelling of lymph through lymphatic vessels. Exercising causes muscles to contract and relax, which propels fluid through the vessels and pulls it away from the tissues. Because exercise is considered a stimulant for lymph circulation, inactivity would therefore be a hindrance to circulation.

Edema

Edema is a condition where excess fluid saturates tissues. There is a buildup, or overload of lymphatic flow, that leads to swelling. Edema can be contributed to overconsumption of salt or fluids, a sedentary lifestyle, or scar tissue blocking lymphatic flow in the case of minor injuries.

There are two types of edema: primary lymphedema (a congenital malformation of blood and lymph vessels) and secondary lymphedema (an obstruction in the lymph system caused by infection, injury, or surgery). In both cases, the tissue fluid cannot be removed because of this blockage, and the fluid therefore becomes stagnate and can lead to bacterial growth, stagnate proteins that may be treated as foreign invaders. The cycle brought on by chronic stagnate fluid can result in inflammation, pain, heat, and redness, and ultimately the tissues may scar, leading to a cycle of more edema. Chronic edema leads to chronic inflammation and fibrosis that makes tissues coarser, thicker, less flexible, and tender. Severe cases can lead to lymphedema. **Obstructive lymphedema** is caused by scar tissue that can cause blockage and is commonly seen in elephantiasis (a parasite infects the lymphatics, leaving scar tissue) or with surgery and radiation therapy that also scars the tissues. It is common for lymphedema to occur after cancer treatment. Other causes include heart and kidney disease; certain medications, like steroids and hormone therapy; chemotherapy; and allergic reactions and muscle tension caused by stress. When working with a client who has obstructive edema, there are some standards to follow. Begin the treatment sequence by addressing the unaffected side then moving to the affected side. For edema due to obstructions in the lower body, focus on the inguinal nodes, and for upper body edema, focus on the cervical and axillary nodes.

obstructive lymphedema
swelling of tissues with lymph stasis

Watersheds

Watersheds are the areas of division between each of the four quadrants of the body that divide the lymph system. There are two watersheds, the medial sagittal watershed (a vertical division of the body) and the transverse watershed (dividing the body horizontally around the waist area), that divide the trunk into four quadrants. Because of the watersheds, lymph can be directed around obstructions and drained toward the nodes of the unaffected side of the body. The lymph system needs to be stimulated on the unaffected side so that it can carry the lymph from the obstructed side to the lymph nodes for cleansing.

watersheds
drainage divide or the area that separates or divides two drainage basins

stationary circle
light form of circular massage using the fingertips

Physiological Effects of Manual or Machine Assisted Lymphatic Drainage

Lymphatic drainage helps to open up the initial lymphatics and stimulate lymph vessel contraction. This moves fluid out of the body tissue and into the lymph system where it can be cleansed and purified by the lymph nodes and the lymphocytes. It also stimulates a parasympathetic reaction that slows heart rate, relaxes muscles, and allows organs to resume normal function, thereby reducing stress levels.

Pressure and Movement

The basis of the drainage technique is the **stationary circle**, performed with a circular motion while remaining stationary. This movement involves a slight compression followed by a stretch of tissue. If you draw a circle and divide it in half, consider one half the "on pressure" and the other half the "off or zero pressure." (See Figure 6–3.) As a result of this on/off pressure, the lymph capillaries are stretched in different directions, which cause them to contract and stimulate the lymphatic system. Pressure during the process should be gentle, and a focus on moving the upper epidermal areas will provide a good baseline. The rate of massage should be the same as the rate at which lymphatics contract. Massage strokes should therefore start out at a rate of one stroke every 10 seconds, slow and rhythmic, with a direction of movement toward the lymph nodes.

Sequence

Lymph nodes should be cleared at the beginning of the lymphatic drainage session in order to allow the lymphatic fluid to flow freely. Because lymph circulation slows at the lymph nodes, excess fluid is likely

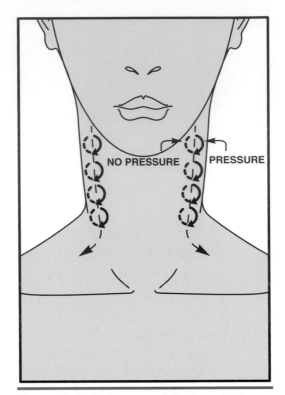

Figure 6–3 A diagram of the lymphatic drainage technique for the neck area

to accumulate if the nodes are not properly drained. During the session, a large amount of fluid will be moved to the lymph nodes. It is therefore important to massage the nodes at the conclusion of the process to avoid edema. If you are performing a neck and face sequence you will want to clear the nodes of the neck first, then perform the face drainage techniques, and conclude with a final draining sequence to the neck. When performing drainage to the face and body, you will perform a clearing of the neck before the draining of the body and face, and end with a clearing of the neck. It is imperative to pay attention to subtle changes in the temperature, the texture, and the elasticity of the tissue to help you visualize the movement of the lymph through the tissues. Successful treatments can only be achieved through focus and concentration.

Health Screening

Records should include a client's health history and activity level, goals and expectations, concerns you may have, and any contraindications. It is important to find out the cause for edema before performing a treatment, and a physician must rule out serious conditions before treatment can be performed. During the initial visit, procedures and outcomes should be explained to the client. The beginning of each session starts out with light effleurage, to desensitize the skin. The end of treatment involves a firmer effleurage to indicate to the client the session is ending. Advise the client to drink water, as it is important for the client to flush the body posttreatment. After the treatment, note any important observations; it may also be helpful to have a chart with locations of the lymph nodes to log any specific data.

General Indications and Contraindications

Lymphatic drainage can speed healing and reduce swelling caused by injury or surgery, reduce scar tissue, improve the health and appearance of the skin, help treat cellulite, stimulate a sluggish immune system, reduce stress and tension, and relax the muscles.

Lymphatic drainage should not be performed immediately following surgery or an injury.

Absolute contraindications following soft tissue injury and surgery include:

- blood clots
- open wounds and abnormal drainage
- heart disease and congestive heart failure
- fevers and chronic infections
- kidney failure and kidney dialysis
- allergic reactions
- varicose veins that are hot, red, swollen, painful

It is important to consult a physician in the following cases:

- chronic edema
- cancer patients
  - chemotherapy
  - radiation
- phlebitis
- organ transplants

It is never advisable to perform lymph drainage on anyone who is sick or beginning to feel unwell.

Treatment Focal Areas

The densest population of lymph nodes occurs in the head and neck region because disease-causing organisms can easily enter through the mouth, nose, and eyes. The face and neck treatment will stimulate the circulation of the facial and cervical lymph nodes. This can help reduce swelling and bruising, stimulate a sluggish immune system, improve fatigue, and improve the skin by eliminating excess toxins in the tissues and allowing nutrients to flow into the skin. Aestheticians incorporate lymphatic drainage into facial treatments in place of the massage to achieve greater results, or they may employ lymphatic drainage as a stand-alone treatment. Eye treatments may also include the use of lymphatic drainage to help with dark circles and swollen and puffy eyes. Many European women rely on the use of lymphatic drainage during pregnancy for swollen or tired legs, and lymphatic drainage is a staple of cellulite treatments.

Lymphatic drainage may also be performed to elevate edema that may have resulted from injury, an obstruction from surgery, or scar tissue. Because blood clots can be a possibility, any client with edema that is red, hot, and painful should see a physician before receiving any treatment. Many preoperative patients also use lymphatic drainage to help prepare for surgery, and postoperatively it will speed healing by reducing edema and by stimulating the immune system. Postoperative lymphatic drainage must be cleared with the acting physician and must be performed with care not to disrupt any sutures.

■ PATTERNS OF LYMPH FLOW

When discussing general lymph flow starting at the head and moving to the lower limbs, lymph from the crown and the posterior portion of the head drains to the occipital nodes. Superficial lymph fluid located in the head area drains to the lymph nodes in the neck. Lymph from the facial area drains toward the preauricular and mandibular nodes and then flows into the cervical nodes. The right arm and trunk drain to the right axillary nodes. The left arm and trunk drain to the left axillary nodes. The lymph from the sternum drains to the nodes located in the neck area. Superficial lymph from the lower left portion of the body drains to the left inguinal nodes. Superficial lymph from the lower right portion of the body drains to the right inguinal nodes.

The lymph nodes in the upper quadrants of the body include the central axillary nodes, the pectoral nodes, the subscapular nodes, the lateral nodes, the infraclavicular nodes, the supraclavicular nodes, and the internal mammary chain nodes. When discussing the drainage patterns of the upper quadrant, lymph drains from the chest into the pectoral, subscapular, and lateral nodes, into the central axillary nodes, and up to the infraclavicular and supraclavicular nodes.

The lymph nodes in the lower quadrants are in the femoral triangle, the inguinal ligament, and the sartorius and adductor muscles. Two chains of lymph nodes, the horizontal and superior chains, are located near the inguinal ligament and the femoral vein. The popliteal nodes are located near the middle of the knee. When discussing the drainage patterns of the upper quadrant, lymph drains from the lower back and abdomen around the hips to the inguinal nodes. Drainage from the back of the thighs is around the front and up to the inguinal nodes. The inguinal nodes are inferior to the inguinal ligament in a depression of muscles where the femoral triangle is.

You should begin the lymphatic drainage session by checking the nodes for asymmetry or swelling before proceeding. Begin by palpating the lymph nodes, and massage over the areas using small circles where lymph nodes are located, feeling for pea-sized masses. (Lymph nodes on a healthy person are small and typically cannot be felt.)

■ "DRAINAGETHERAPY" MANUAL LYMPHATIC DRAINAGE TREATMENT

Lymphatic drainage is performed on both sides of the face and neck at the same time. The most common massage movement is the stationary circle. With the following sequence outlined below you will not have to drain the back areas of the client.

■ MACHINE AIDED LYMPHATIC DRAINAGE TREATMENTS

Once found only in Europe, a popular lymphatic drainage machine that made its way to the United States is called pressotherapy. The pressotherapy equipment is composed of a compression system designed to increase the venous and lymphatic flow and enhance extracellular fluid clearance. Pressotherapy equipment includes a computer-controlled pump that inflates the individual sections of the multichambered garments. The garment has five separate chambers, which are positioned around the limbs. The chambers focus on moving the venous and lymph flow, starting from the ankles and moving to the upper thighs. The pump inflates each chamber of the garment individually as well as in a preset sequence and time period, according to predetermined parameters. Pressotherapy also reduces bloating, swelling, and edema, alleviates

Suggested Steps for Lymphatic Drainage

NECK

1. Divide the neck in half, just to the left and right of the trachea. Define three horizontal lines on each side of the neck beginning medial and moving lateral (inward and moving to the outside of the neck). The innermost line will be defined as line 1, the middle line, line 2, and the outermost line, line 3. On the first defined line, begin using stationary circles, moving superior to inferior (top, just under the jawline to bottom, the base of the neck). (You will separate your hands and perform stationary circles on line 1 on both sides of the neck at the same time.) The number of circles you will perform on each line will be related to the length of the neck; an average is three. Repeat three to five times. Moving lateral (outward), move to the second defined line. Moving superior to inferior (top to bottom) on defined line 2, begin using stationary circles. Repeat three to five times. Moving lateral (outward), move to the third defined line and begin using stationary circles, moving superior to inferior (top to bottom). Repeat three to five times.

2. Place your hands on the base of the skull behind the neck. Define one line down the spinal column and move just slightly to the left and right and begin using stationary circles, moving superior to inferior. Repeat three to five times on this same defined line.

3. Repeat the same moves as in step one and add the following downward draining movements at the conclusion: On lines 1, 2, and 3 at the same time, use a draining stroke (gliding stroke using gentle and superficial pressure of your pointer, middle, and ring finger tips) to drain fluid from the jawline to the base of the neck. Repeat three to five times and end with a stationary circle drain on the back of the neck at the base, closest to the shoulder area.

4. On lines 1, 2, and 3 at the same time, use an openhanded, pumping motion (butterfly-like movement) with the pointer, middle, and ring finger tips to drain fluid from the base of the neck moving up to the jawline. Repeat three to five times and end with a stationary circle drain on the back of the neck at the base, closest to the shoulder area.

5. On the clavicle (on bone) moving medial to lateral (outer to inward) perform stationary circles on the bone. Just below the clavicle bone (inferior) moving medial to lateral (outer to inward) perform stationary circles just below the bone. Repeat three to five times.

6. Separate your hands and place them on the clavicle bone at the points closest to the shoulder. Separate the fingers on your hand to a position where your ring and middle fingers are straddling the clavicle bone. Working from a lateral to medial position on the bone, use the ring and middle fingers to perform a stretch press draining motion. (The number of press/drain points you will perform on each line will be related to the length of the clavicle bone; an average is three to four points.) Repeat three to five times.

FACE

1. Begin with both hands fully open, touching together with your pointer fingers anchored on the sides of the nose. Begin to rock your hands from palm to back of hand while descending from the cheek to the nose area and to the ear area up and back down again. This will produce a butterfly-like movement. Repeat three to five times.

2. Separate both hands and begin with the hands anchored in a claw-type stance on the mandible (on the area just under the chin), moving laterally toward the mastoid process (near ear area). (Perform stationary circles chin to jaw.) Repeat three to five times.

3. Beginning at the middle of the chin, take your thumb and pointer finger and press the outline of the chin to the jaw area as if you are performing a draining movement. Repeat three to five times.

4. Beginning at the middle of the chin take your thumb and alternate thumb over thumb movements along the upper chin area just below the lower lip, eventually moving upward to cover the upper lip area just below the nose. Perform as if you are performing a draining movement. Repeat three to five times.

5. Beginning on the chin just below the lower lip, use your middle and pointer fingers to perform an alternating hand over hand movement as if you are performing a draining movement, guiding the fluids to the outer facial areas. Repeat three to five times.

6. Beginning on the chin just below the lower lip, use your middle or thumb finger to perform a simultaneous sweeping movement as if you are guiding the fluids to the outer facial areas. Slowly move upward, covering the upper lip area just under the nose. Repeat three to five times.

7. Separate your hands and anchor them gently on both sides of the outer lips. Perform stationary circles with your pointer and middle fingers. Repeat three to five times.

8. Returning to the middle chin area just below the lower lip, use your middle and pointer fingers to perform an alternating hand over hand movement as if you are performing a draining movement, guiding the fluids to the outer facial areas. Slowly move upward, covering the upper lip area just under the nose. Repeat three to five times.

9. Separate your hands and anchor them gently on both sides of the base of the nose. Using your pointer and middle fingers, perform stationary circles. Repeat three to five times.

10. Separate your hands and anchor them gently on both sides of the top of the nose (near the lacrimal bone). Using your pointer and middle fingers, perform stationary circles. Repeat three to five times.

11. Using your pointer and middle fingers, perform stationary circles moving from the top of the nose to the base (nostril area). Repeat three to five times.

12. Visualize an imaginary line from the base of the nose diagonal outwards toward the ear (following the temporal process of the zygomatic bone). Separate your hands and anchor them gently on both sides of the bottom of the nose (nostril area) and perform stationary circles moving from the nose outward toward the ear area. Using your pointer and middle fingers, perform stationary circles. Repeat three to five times.

13. On the same line, using a piano tapping movement (pinkie to thumb), move from the nose to outer ear area. Repeat three to five times.

14. Begin with stationary circles on the temple area and move along the exterior portion of the face, descending down the jawline. Repeat three to five times.

15. Use the butterfly movement with the palm of the hand on the outer cheek, working up toward the nose area and back down again. Repeat three to five times.

(Continued)

16. Beginning at the middle of the nose, just under the eye, and moving out to the temple area, take your thumbs and alternate (separated hand and work both sides of the face simultaneously), with draining movements as to drain fluid from the cheek area to hairline. Repeat three to five times. Repeat three to five times.

17. Beginning at the middle of the forehead just slightly above the brow line, moving out to the temple area, take your thumb and alternate (separate hand and work both sides of the face simultaneously), with draining movements as to drain fluid from the brow line area to the hairline. Repeat three to five times. Repeat three to five times.

18. Beginning at the medial end of one brow, work toward the end of the brow using a gentle pinching movement (as if you are draining fluid to the hairline) and inch along the brow line until you reach the tail end of the brow. Repeat three to five times. Now perform the same steps on the other brow. Repeat three to five times.

19. With both thumbs between the brows, following the brow or the area just above the brow line, perform an alternating draining movement as if you are guiding the fluids to the outer facial areas. Repeat three to five times.

20. With the pointer and middle fingers between the brows, walk the fingers upward, alternating between the middle and pointer fingers, walking the fingers upward to the middle of the forehead, performing a draining movement as if you are guiding the fluids to the upper forehead regions. Repeat three to five times.

21. With both thumbs between the brows, following the brow or the area just above the brow line, perform an alternating draining movement as if you are guiding the fluids to the outer facial areas. Repeat three to five times.

22. Place the palms of the hands on the forehead and alternate hand over hand while using draining movements as if to drain the fluid from the forehead down the temples to the cheek area. Work one side and then the other. Repeat three to five times.

23. Use the butterfly movement with the palm of the hand on the outer cheek, working up toward the nose area and back down again, to drain the fluids from the temple to the cheeks back down to the neck area. Repeat three to five times. End by working from the forehead and perform the butterfly motions again back down to the neck area. Repeat three to five times.

24. An optional move of effleurage or vibration may be used in the closing of the face section.

25. Conclude the face and neck sequence by repeating the neck sequence again. If you are proceeding to perform the sequence on the entire body, you will perform the neck sequence at the end of the body sequence.

LEG

1. Define one diagonal line along the inguinal nodes (bikini line area); using stationary circles move lateral to medial until you reach the inner thigh region. Repeat three to five times.

2. Along the same diagonal line along the inguinal nodes (bikini line area) with one hand on top of the other hand, use the heel of the hand to the tip of the finger to produce a wave-like motion to

systematically inch your way from the top of the leg down to the inner thigh area. Repeat three to five times.

3. Divide the leg into three horizontal zones running from the top of the thigh to mid thigh (zone 1), from the mid thigh to lower thigh (zone 2), and from the lower thigh to knee area (zone 3). (You will begin by draining zone 1, then 2, and then 3.) Beginning at the upper thigh area, working down to knee area, sweep and scoop your hands from the inner and outer thigh up together (simultaneously) to the top of the leg. Move down to zone 2 and scoop and sweep from inner and outer thigh up to the top of the leg and push both hands up as if you are pressing fluid up to the top of the thigh with the heel of your hand and the upper arm area (passing zone 1). Move down to zone 3 and scoop and sweep from inner and outer thigh up to the top of the leg and push both hands up as if you are pressing fluid up to the top of the thigh with the heel of your hand and the upper arm area (passing zone 2 and zone 1). Repeat three to five times.

4. Beginning in zone 3, scoop and sweep from inner and outer thigh up to the top of the leg and push both hands up as if you are pressing fluid up to the top of the thigh with the heel of your hand and the upper arm area (passing zone 2 and zone 1). Repeat three to five times.

5. Separate hands, placing both hands under the knee area side by side, and use stationary circles to drain the popliteal lymph node. Repeat 12 to 15 times.

6. Divide the lower portion of the leg (knee to ankle) into three horizontal zones running from the bottom of the knee to the mid calf area (zone 1), from the mid calf to the lower calf (zone 2), and from the lower calf to the ankle area (zone 3). You will begin by draining zone 1, then 2, and then 3. Beginning at the area just below the knee, working down to the ankle area, sweep and scoop your hands from the outer sides of the mid calf area (simultaneously) to the top of the knee and press through to just above the knee. Move down to zone 2 and scoop and sweep from inner and outer mid calf, pushing both hands up as if you are pressing fluid up to the top of the leg with the heel of your hand and the upper arm area (passing zone 1). Move down to zone 3 and scoop and sweep from inner and outer lower calf area up to the top of the leg, and push both hands up as if you are pressing fluid up to the top of the leg just past the knee with the heel of your hand and the upper arm area (passing zone 2 and zone 1). Repeat three to five times.

7. Beginning in zone 3, scoop and sweep from inner and outer lower leg area (ankle area) up to the top of the leg and push both hands up as if you are pressing fluid up to the top of the leg, just past the knee with the heel of your hand and upper arm area (passing zone 2 and zone 1). Repeat three to five times.

8. In the foot area you will use a pumping or rocking motion to drain the toes. Divide the toes into three zones including tip, middle, and base (where the toe is attached to the foot). Using your thumbs on both hands, grasp two toes at a time and begin to pump tip to middle to base, in a rocking motion from middle of thumb to tip to press and drain the fluid. Repeat three to five times. Repeat until all five toes on the foot are completed.

9. Using the pointer, ring, and middle fingers placed under the foot, with the thumbs of the hands on top, begin a pressing movement from the base of the toes moving toward the heel of the foot, draining fluid toward the ankle area. Repeat three to five times.

(Continued)

10. Divide the top of the foot into three zones. Imagine three horizontal lines that run along the foot from the base of the toes to the ankle (there you will notice tendons that run along this area, and between the tendons are grooves that the fingers will easily fall into). Use the thumbs to press and slightly pump simultaneously to drain toward the ankle. Move from lateral to medial (small toe to large toe). Repeat three to five times.

11. Separate hands, placing both hands on either side of the ankle, and use stationary circles to drain the ankle area. Repeat 12 to 15 times.

12. Beginning in zone 3 (ankle area), scoop and sweep from inner and outer lower leg area (ankle area) up to the top of the leg and push both hands up as if you are pressing fluid up to the top of the leg, just past the knee with the heel of your hand and the upper arm area (passing zone 2 and zone 1). Repeat three to five times.

13. Beginning in zone 3 (ankle area), press the sides of the legs and push upward from inner and outer lower leg area (ankle area) up to the top of the leg and push both hands up as if you are pressing fluid up to the top of the leg, just past the knee with the heel of your hand and the upper arm area (passing zone 2 and zone 1). Repeat three to five times. Optional: A wave-like motion may be used or a movement similar to wringing performed on the inner and alternating to the outer area, moving from the ankle to the knee area.

14. Raise the knee to a bent position and begin by clearing out the back of the ankle. Separate hands, placing both hands on either side of the ankle, and use stationary circles to drain the ankle area. Repeat 12 to 15 times.

15. Working on the back of the lower leg area only, begin in zone 3 (ankle area), pump and press the back side of the legs and push upward from the ankle area up to the top of the leg. Using both hands around the back of the leg, push both hands up as if you are pressing fluid up to the top of the leg, just past the knee with the heel of your hand and the upper arm area (passing zone 2 and zone 1) on the lower leg past zones 1, 2, and 3 on the upper portion of the leg. Repeat three to five times.

16. Working on the back of the upper leg area only, begin in zone 3 (lower thigh to knee area); using both hands around the back of the leg, push both hands up as if you are pressing fluid up to the top of the leg, just past the mid thigh with the heel of your hand and the upper arm area (passing zone 2 and zone 1) on the upper leg. Progressively move up to zone 2 and repeat and move to zone 1 and repeat. Repeat three to five times.

17. With knee still bent, begin back down in zone 3 (ankle area) and move up and over the knee, to zone 1 of the upper thigh. Push both hands up as if you are pressing fluid up to the top of the leg, just past the mid thigh with the heel of your hand and the upper arm area (passing zone 2 and zone 1) on the upper leg. Repeat three to five times.

18. Separate hands, placing both hands under the knee area side by side, and use stationary circles to drain the popliteal lymph node. Repeat 12 to 15 times.

19. Beginning at the lower thigh area, moving upward to the middle thigh area (zone 3), sweep and scoop your hands from the inner and outer thigh up together (simultaneously) to the top of the leg. Move up to zone 2 and scoop and sweep from the inner and outer thigh up to the top of the leg and push both hands up as if you are pressing fluid up to the top of the thigh with the heel of your

hand and the upper arm area (passing zone 1). Move up to zone 1 and scoop and sweep from the inner and outer thigh up to the top of the leg and push both hands up as if you are pressing fluid up to the top of the thigh with the heel of your hand and upper arm area (passing zone 2 and zone 1). Repeat three to five times.

20. Beginning in zone 3, scoop and sweep from inner and outer lower leg area (ankle area) up to the top of the leg and push both hands up as if you are pressing fluid up to the top of the leg, just past the knee with the heel of your hand and the upper arm area (passing zone 2 and zone 1). An alternative move would be a wave-like motion or a movement similar to wringing performed on the inner and alternating to the outer area, moving from the lower thigh to the upper thigh area. Repeat three to five times.

21. Divide the upper leg into three zones consisting of horizontal lines, zone 1 being outer thigh, zone 2 inner thigh, and zone 3 top of the thigh. Perform stationary circles, moving from the lower thigh to upper thigh. Repeat on zones 2 and 3. Repeat three to five times.

22. Beginning in zone 3, scoop and sweep from inner and outer thigh to the upper thigh area and push both hands up as if you are pressing fluid up to the top of the leg (passing zone 2 and zone 1). An alterative move would be a wave-like motion or a movement similar to wringing performed on the inner thigh and alternating to the outer thigh.

23. As in the beginning, define one diagonal line along the inguinal nodes (bikini line area). Using stationary circles move lateral to medial until you reach the inner thigh region. Repeat three to five times.

24. Repeat on the other side from start to finish.

ABDOMINAL AREA

1. Divide the umbilical region of the abdominal area in half. Beginning on the left side of the body, moving around the umbilicus (navel area), perform stationary circles. The circles will be performed with one hand directly on top of the other (double handed method). Move directly on top of the umbilicus and perform stationary circles. Repeat each stationary circle three to five times.

2. Move to the right lumbar region, perform stationary circles, and then move across the upper hypogastric region to the left lumbar region. Repeat each stationary circle three to five times.

3. Separate your hands and begin stationary circles on the back area on the right lumbar and left lumbar regions. Repeat each stationary circle three to five times.

4. Continuing to use a hand on hand position, begin to palpitate the left lumbar region into the umbilical region. Repeat three to five times. Repeat on the other side.

5. Place both hands side by side with the thumbs together in a "V" position, with the umbilical region inside the "V" and palpitate upward. Repeat each palpitation three to five times.

6. Move above the umbilical region to the epigastric region and palpitate from left to right. Repeat each palpitation three to five times.

BREAST AREA

1. Move up the sternum toward the clavicle area performing double handed (one on top of another) stationary circles. Repeat each circle three to five times.

(Continued)

2. When at the clavicle area above the left breast over the heart area, perform double handed stationary circles. Repeat each circle three to five times.

3. Just below the lower left breast, perform a palpitating double handed motion medial to lateral. Repeat each palpitation three to five times.

4. Just below the lower right breast, perform a palpitating double handed motion medial to lateral. Repeat each palpitation three to five times.

5. When at the clavicle area above the right breast over the heart area, perform double handed stationary circles moving lateral to medial (outer to inner). Repeat each circle three to five times.

6. Palpitate just above the fold of the right arm and then left. Repeat each palpitation three to five times.

ARM AREA

1. Raise the arm above the head; use stationary circles in areas of the axillary nodes moving superior to inferior. Repeat each circle three to five times.

2. Continue using stationary circles, working from the upper axillary area to the elbow area. Repeat each circle three to five times.

3. Lift arm up and support the hand against your abdomen. Separate hands, placing hands on each side of the elbow, and use thumbscrew-like, stationary circles to drain the elbow area. Repeat 12 to 15 times.

4. Use the heel of your hand, rocking to the tips of your fingers to pump and drain toward the axillary area. Repeat each pump three to five times.

5. Lower the arm into anatomical position and, using one hand, press and push from the elbow region up to the upper shoulder region. Repeat sequence three to five times.

6. Separate hands, placing one on the bottom side of the elbow, and use thumbscrew-like, stationary circles to drain the elbow area. Repeat 12 to 15 times.

7. Using one hand, press and push from the wrist joint region up to the elbow region. Repeat sequence three to five times.

8. On the hand, you will use a pumping or rocking motion to drain the fingers. Divide the fingers into three zones including tip, middle, and base (where finger is attached to the hand). Using your thumbs on both hands, grasp two fingers at a time and begin to pump tip to middle to base, in a rocking motion from middle of thumb to tip to press and drain the fluid. Repeat three to five times. Repeat until all five fingers are completed.

9. Using the pointer, ring, and middle fingers placed under the hand, with the thumbs of the hands on top of the client's hand, begin a pressing movement from the base of the hand moving toward the wrist area. Repeat three to five times.

10. Divide the top of the hand into three zones. Imagine three horizontal lines that run along the hand from the base of the fingers to the wrist (there you will notice tendons that run along this area, and between the tendons are grooves that the fingers will easily fall into). Use the thumbs to press and slightly pump simultaneously to drain toward the wrist. Move from lateral to medial (small toe to large toe). Repeat three to five times.

11. Separate hands, placing both hands on either side of the clients hand and use thumbscrew-like motions working from the base of the fingers to the wrist and drain toward the wrist. Repeat three to five times. Continue this motion up the arm to the elbow region. Begin again at the wrist area, working upward with one hand only, and continue up and over the elbow to the shoulder area. Repeat three to five times.

12. Separate both hands and begin at the wrist area, sweeping from the outer regions of the arm up and together to meet at the elbow region, continuing up and over and up toward the shoulder. Repeat three to five times.

13. Brace the client's hand in yours, bend the arm at the elbow, and place your hands so they encircle the lower area. Starting at the wrist and moving toward the elbow, press downwards as if you are draining fluid toward the elbow. Repeat three to five times.

14. While still bracing the client's arm, take your other hand and palpitate the axilla area. Repeat three to five times.

15. Repeat on the other arm.

If you are draining the body areas only, begin with the neck sequence, then perform the full body sequence, and end with the neck sequence again. If you are draining the face and body areas, perform the neck sequence, the face sequence, and the full body sequence, and end with the neck sequence.

leg fatigue, and improves oxygen flow through the whole body. Pressotherapy can be used in conjunction with seaweed wraps to detoxify, firm, tone, improve circulation, and increase lymphatic drainage. Pressotherapy is very popular in Europe and is usually associated with cellulite treatments.

A typical vacuum or suction lymphatic drainage machine will have a push-pull action, achieved with a computer-controlled pump or compressor. Some manufacturers will have a machine specifically made to achieve these results, but a typical vacuum apparatus (on a multifunction machine) combined with a rhythmic tapping (on/off action) on the vacuum hole of the glass attachment will achieve the same results. The intensity of the vacuum apparatus will need to be set at low for face and neck areas and medium to low for deeper seated lymphatics or body work. Some companies make larger bell-shaped glass suction cups that can easily be adapted to the multifunction machine to mimic expensive lymphatic drainage machines.

The vacuum or suction action will mimic the contractions made within the lymph vessels and assist with the movement of the lymphatic fluid. Many therapists find that using these machines will allow them to treat more clients in a day than is possible with laborious manual methods of lymphatic drainage. Others argue that the machines are not as effective as manual therapies, and there has been much discussion over this debate.

Example of an Intake Form to Use in Practice

Lymphatic Drainage Massage

Date _____

Name _____

Address _____

Phone _____ DOB _____

Do you have any of the following conditions: kidney failure _____ phlebitis _____

congestive heart failure _____ blood clots _____ heart disease _____cancer _____

List any allergies you have: _____

List any skin disorders you have: _____

Identify the location of any of the following:

      sunburn _____

      acne _____

      abnormal drainage _____

      open wounds _____

      infections _____

      varicose veins _____

      scar tissue _____

      fractures/sprains _____

List any medications you are currently taking: _____

Are you currently receiving chemotherapy or radiation treatment? _____

Have you ever had an organ transplant?_____

Are you on your menstrual cycle? _____

Are you pregnant? _____

What are you hoping to achieve from lymphatic drainage massage?_____

I understand it is my responsibility to notify the technician of any changes to this information.

Signature _____

Scientific studies tend to lean toward greater effectiveness with manual therapy, but as with anything it is dependant on the skill and knowledge of the therapist.

▪ CELLULITE

cellulite
dimpling of the skin caused by the protrusion of subcutaneous fat

Cellulite appears as dimpled or bumpy skin, is due to an irregularity in the distribution of fat in the area, and is commonly found on the thighs, buttocks, and abdomen. Cellulite forms in the superficial fascia, the layer of connective tissue below the skin that contains fat cells. Cellulite should be viewed not as fat accumulation but as imbalances that lead to structural disturbances. Cellulite is more prevalent in females and can be linked to

Example of a Brochure that Explains the Benefits of LDM to Your Clients

Lymphatic Drainage Massage

- Are you frequently ill?
- Do you have extensive recovery periods from illness?
- Do you lack energy and feel sluggish?
- Do you have poor circulation?
- Do you experience chronic swelling?
- Would you like to improve your skins overall health and appearance?

LDM May Be Able To Help You!

What is LDM?

Lymphatic Drainage Massage (LDM) is a gentle style of massage that mimics the action of the lymphatic system that distributes immune cells throughout the body, filters waste out of the blood system, and repairs tissues.

What can LDM treat?

- LDM can speed healing and reduce swelling caused by injury or surgery
- LDM can reduce scar tissue
- LDM can improve the health and appearance of your skin
- LDM can help treat cellulite
- LDM can stimulate a sluggish immune system
- LDM can energize the body
- LDM can reduce stress and tension
- LDM can relax the muscles

What does LDM do?

Lymphatic Drainage Massage (LDM) stimulates the lymphatic system. The lymphatic system is responsible for cleaning out the bloodstream by directing the blood to the lymph nodes. The lymph nodes filter out impurities and waste material so that clean blood can be redirected to tissues. This oxygenates the tissues and washes away impurities that are once again sent to the lymph nodes for purification.

How can LDM help?

Stimulating the lymphatic system stimulates the immune system. The immune system is responsible for destroying the bacterial invaders in your body that cause illness. When the immune system is circulating properly, your body is better protected from disease and illness. This improves your overall health, which you will feel on the inside, and this will show on the outside.

(*Continued*)

The absolute LDM contraindications immediately after soft tissue injury and surgery

LDM should not be performed immediately following surgery or an injury.

Absolute contraindications following soft tissue injury and surgery include:

- blood clots
- open wounds and abnormal drainage
- heart disease and congestive heart failure
- fevers and chronic infections
- kidney failure and kidney dialysis
- allergic reactions
- varicose veins that are hot, red, swollen, painful

When the therapist consults the client's physician before giving a massage

It is important to consult a physician in the following cases:

- chronic edema
- cancer patients
  - chemotherapy
  - radiation
- phlebitis
- organ transplants

falling estrogen levels, genetic predisposition, hormone imbalances, and disruptions in microcirculation. Lymph drainage and microcirculation are particularly affected, resulting in an accumulation of toxins, cellular by-products, and metabolic waste and causing alterations in connective tissue and the fat cells, which are held in a framework of the collagen fiber network. Through this long term imbalance, fat cells that are displaced can migrate upwards into the lower dermis. Dislodged or damaged portions of fibrous bands that normally maintain skin tension trap the displaced cells. The "cottage cheese" appearance is caused by the restriction of fibrous strands as they pull down the skin at their attachment points that are still intact. If this process is left unhindered, further hardening or developments of micronodules are prevalent and further lead to larger macronodules. Development of hard fibrous tissues and macronodules are noted with more advanced stages of cellulite. With advanced stages of cellulite, the affected area will become very painful and very visible to the naked eye. These changes can be compared to a change from an orange peel appearance to a cottage cheese appearance of the skin and tissues.

As discussed earlier, in Europe, many women used lymphatic drainage as a method to combat cellulite. Manual or machine modalities (endermologie or vacuum suction machines combined with bipolar

Suggested Steps for Machine Assisted Lymphatic Drainage with Vacuum Machines

(1) Begin with light effleurage movements.

(2) Have the client turn the face to one side and place the handpiece on the postauricular area (behind the ear under the hairline). Move the handpiece down the neck to the clavicle. Repeat the sequence three to five times. Repeat sequence on the other side of the neck, three to five times.

(3) Have the client straighten the head to supine position.

(4) Separate handpieces so that you have one in each hand. Place the handpieces just below the preauricular area (in front of the ear) and move downwards to the clavicle. Repeat the sequence three to five times.

(5) Separate handpieces so that you have one in each hand. Place the handpieces on the submental area (under the jaw) and move downwards to the clavicle. Repeat until you have cleared the front of the neck, but exclude the trachea area. Repeat the sequence three to five times.

(6) Separate handpieces so that you have one in each hand. Place the handpieces so that they are touching side by side on the top of the chin just above the submental area (above the jawline) and move downwards to the clavicle. Repeat the sequence three to five times.

(7) Separate handpieces so that you have one in each hand. Place the handpieces so that they are touching side by side on the top of the lip, just below the nose, move out to the ear area, and continue to move downwards to the clavicle. Repeat the sequence three to five times.

(8) Separate handpieces so that you have one in each hand. Place the handpieces on both sides of the face so that they are level with the top of the ears, and move downwards to the jawline. Repeat the sequence three to five times.

(9) Separate handpieces so that you have one in each hand. Place the handpieces on either side of the nose, move out to the ear area, and continue to move downwards to the jawline. Repeat until you have moved progressively up to the area just under the eye. Typically this can be achieved with three points. Repeat the sequence three to five times.

(10) Separate handpieces so that you have one in each hand. Place the handpieces just under the eye, gently move out to the ear area, and continue to move out to the corners of the eye and to the lower temple area. Repeat the sequence three to five times.

(11) Separate handpieces so that you have one in each hand. Place the handpieces on the brow line, and move out to the temple area. Repeat the sequence three to five times.

(12) Separate handpieces so that you have one in each hand. Place the handpieces on the forehead just above the brows, move outwards to the hairline, and continue to move downwards to the temples. Repeat until you have cleared the middle forehead and upper forehead areas. Repeat the sequence three to five times.

(13) Separate handpieces so that you have one in each hand. Place the handpieces superior on either side of the temple, continue to move downwards to the jawline, and proceed to the clavicle. Repeat the sequence three to five times. End the face and neck sequence by repeating the neck area as follows: Have the client turn the face to one side and place the handpiece on the postauricular area (behind the ear, under the hairline). Move the handpiece down the neck to the clavicle. Repeat the sequence three to five times. Repeat the sequence on the other side of the neck, three to five times.

(14) End with light effleurage movements.

Stages of Cellulite

Stage 1: The skin will show no visible signs of cellulite. When pinched the skin shows slight "orange-peel" effect.

Stage 2: The skin will show no visible signs, except for when sitting or crossing legs. When pinched the skin shows definite orange-peel effect.

Stage 3: The skin will show a definite orange-peel appearance without pinching the skin.

Stage 4: The skin will show a definite orange-peel appearance without pinching the skin, and large lumps of fat, encased by fibers forming even larger nodules, are present.

radio frequency) will not, however, rearrange the fat deposits but only bring about a change in the appearance. Cellulite creams can help improve the appearance of the skin but are not proven effective at the scientific level. It is believed that, if you determine that you are predisposed to cellulite and you begin to proactively take steps to prevent the initial environment that is conducive to promote this cycle, you will lessen the degree to which you may be affected by cellulite. This is why many young ladies in Europe begin to take care of their bodies with body treatments and lymphatic drainage.

The most effective treatments have combined connective tissue massage and lymphatic drainage. (See Figure 6–4.) Connective tissue massage creates microtears in the superficial fascia that make the tissue longer and

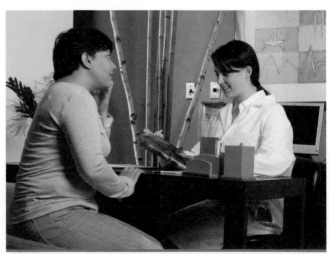

Figure 6–4 Consultations are important before cellulite treatments

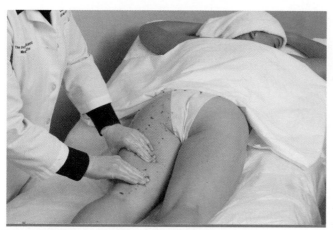

Figure 6–5 An example of a cellulite treatment

more flexible. The superficial fascia can then move more freely and detach itself from underlying structures. These tears will release a trigger for an inflammatory response. Blood flow will increase, bringing nutrition to the tissue and interstitial fluid to cleanse the cells. Lymphatic drainage is then used to stimulate the removal of the interstitial fluid and the toxins it has picked up. These treatments must be employed in a sequence, and client compliance is imperative to achieve the desired results. (See Figure 6–5.) It is also important for the client to become committed to exercise and proper diet, including a reduction in caffeine, sugar, refined carbohydrates, and red meats, as well as an increase in water, fruit, and vegetable intake. Body treatments containing wraps or muds, for an added focus on the appearance of the skin, may also be worked into the treatment protocols.

Suggested Steps for Cellulite Treatments

The consultation is imperative and necessary to determine which type or stage of cellulite is present and which protocols are appropriate to achieve the client's goals.

As previously discussed, a method of deeper massage called skin rolling may be employed. This method involves rolling the skin by picking it up between thumb and fingers and rolling it while walking fingers along, covering the affected region and repeating as necessary. This may be painful initially but will become tolerated by clients as their sessions proceed.

Anticellulite Treatment for Stage One Cellulite (Edematous Phase)

1. On damp skin, carry out a gommage with an exfoliating body treatment or perform a dry brushing.

(Continued)

2. Rinse and dry.

3. Apply the contents of an anticellulite ampoule, followed by the application of an anticellulite cream.

4. Layer an anticellulite mud and leave it in place for 20 minutes, covering the area with a thermal or heated blanket.

5. Rinse and dry.

Complete the treatment with a lymphatic drainage massage or use a pressotherapy treatment machine.

The treatments must be administered in a series of 10 to 15, according to the condition and sensitivity of the skin and the state of development of the cellulite. Monthly maintenance sessions will be required.

Anticellulite Treatment for Stage Two Cellulite (Fibrous Phase)

1. On damp skin, carry out a gommage with an exfoliating body treatment or perform a dry brushing.

2. Rinse and dry.

3. Apply a detoxifying essential oil mixed into a carrier.

4. Apply the contents of an anticellulite ampoule, followed by the application of an anticellulite cream.

5. Layer an anticellulite mud and leave it in place for 20 minutes, covering the area with a thermal or heated blanket.

6. Rinse and dry.

Complete the treatment with a cellulite cream and perform connective tissue massage in the affected areas.

The treatments must be administered in a series of 10 to 15, twice a week. Monthly maintenance sessions will be required

Anticellulite Treatment for Stage Three to Four Cellulite (Advanced Fibrous Phase)
Session 1:

1. On damp skin, carry out a gommage with an exfoliating body treatment or perform a dry brushing.

2. Rinse and dry.

3. Apply a detoxifying essential oil mixed into a carrier.

4. Apply the contents of an anticellulite ampoule, followed by the application of an anticellulite cream.

5. Layer an anticellulite mud and leave in place for 20 minutes, covering the area with a thermal or heated blanket.

6. Rinse and dry.

7. Complete the treatment with a camphor based massage cream and perform connective tissue massage in the affected areas.

Session 2:

1. On damp skin, carry out a gommage with an exfoliating body treatment or perform a dry brushing.

2. Rinse and dry.

3. Apply a detoxifying essential oil mixed into a carrier.

4. Apply the contents of an anticellulite ampoule, followed by the application of an anticellulite cream.

5. Layer an anticellulite mud and leave in place for 20 minutes, covering the area with a thermal or heated blanket.

6. Rinse and dry.

7. Complete the treatment with a drainage massage or use a pressotherapy treatment machine. Complete the treatment with a camphor based massage cream.

Session 3:

1. On damp skin, carry out a gommage with an exfoliating body treatment or perform a dry brushing.

2. Rinse and dry.

3. Apply a detoxifying essential oil mixed into a carrier.

4. Apply the contents of an anticellulite ampoule, followed by the application of an anticellulite cream.

5. Layer an anticellulite mud and leave in place for 20 minutes, covering the area with a thermal or heated blanket.

6. Rinse and dry.

7. Complete the treatment with a camphor based massage cream.

Alternate among session options as desired.

The treatments must be administered in a series of 12 to 18, twice a week. Monthly maintenance sessions are required.

General posttreatment instructions for cellulite treatments

To ensure your client receives the full benefits of this treatment, instruct the client to avoid showering immediately after because the cellulite serums and creams continue to work for several hours. Also stress the importance of rest and replenishing any water loss that has occurred during this treatment. Remind the client to drink plenty of water to continue the detoxification process.

Home-care products can be suggested to maintain the results and are imperative in cellulite treatments. Clients should not take a very hot shower directly after the treatment and should not use harsh exfoliators such as AHAs, BHAs, or other harsh chemicals or cosmetics for 24 to 48 hours after receiving the treatment.

Conclusion

Aestheticians are just beginning to understand the implications of lymphatic drainage and are beginning to implement it as an integral part of face and body treatments. Europeans have employed this technique for years as an integral part of their treatments for the face and body.

Aestheticians can incorporate lymphatic drainage into facial treatments in place of their standard massage. Lymphatic drainage requires advanced training and should not be performed by untrained individuals. Lymphatic drainage is also useful in the treatment of cellulite as well as pre- and postoperatively.

Cellulite appears as dimpled or bumpy skin and is found in more women than men. Cellulite is due to an irregularity in the distribution of fat in the area and is commonly found on the thighs, buttocks, and abdomen due not to obesity but to a breakdown in connective tissues. The fat cells that are held in a framework are displaced and can migrate upwards into the lower dermis. Severe cases of cellulite can be noted by the cottage cheese appearance or the presence of nodules. Cellulite creams can help improve the appearance of the skin but are not proven effective at the scientific level for reducing cellulite itself.

▶ ▷ ▷ TOP 10 TIPS TO TAKE TO THE CLINIC

1. Discuss the risks and benefits of treatments with your client during the consultation.
2. Have your client conduct a thorough health screening.
3. Check for contraindications.
4. Be familiar with treatments or ingredients that are hazardous to certain health conditions.
5. Provide your client with water to drink to prevent dehydration.
6. Provide your client with take-home instructions to maximize the treatment benefits.
7. Offer home-care products to complement the treatments.
8. Prepare your treatment area well ahead of time.
9. Never leave a client unattended during a treatment.
10. Never perform lymphatic drainage treatments on individuals who are sick.

CHAPTER QUESTIONS

1. What is the function of the immune system?
2. What is lymphatic drainage?
3. What are some of the benefits of using lymphatic drainage?
4. What are the contraindications of lymphatic drainage?
5. Provide an example of when lymphatic drainage would be indicated.
6. What is cellulite?
7. What is the purpose of a cellulite treatment?

BIBLIOGRAPHY

Kindt, T. J., Goldsby, R. A., & Osborne, B. A. (2007). *Kuby Immunology*. New York: W. H. Freeman and Company.

Moody French, R. (2004). *Milady's Guide to Lymph Drainage*. Clifton Park, NY: Thomson Delmar Learning.

Exfoliating and Bath Treatments

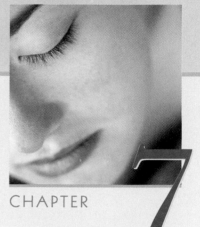

KEY TERMS

alpha hydroxy acids

ayurveda

citric acid

effleurage

exfoliation treatments

fango

fangotherapy

filtration hot springs

footbaths

fruit scrubs

geothermally

glycolic acid

healing baths

lactic acid

malic acid

moor mud

muds

parafango

peat therapy

primary hot springs

salt glow

sea scrub

seaweed baths

sitz bath

watsu

CHAPTER 7

LEARNING OBJECTIVES

After completing this chapter, you should be able to:

1. Describe different types of exfoliating treatment.

2. Discuss different types of mud treatments.

3. Discuss the history of baths.

4. Discuss different types of therapeutic and relaxing baths and their benefits.

5. Discuss different types of water therapy.

6. Discuss steam baths and saunas.

exfoliation treatments
effective for exfoliating the outermost skin cells, revealing a fresh and glowing skin tone

sea scrub
stimulates the circulation, exfoliates the outermost skin cells, moisturizes the skin, and reveals a fresh and glowing skin tone

salt glow
a type of exfoliation process

Exfoliating treatments can be used individually or in preparation for many other body treatments.

INTRODUCTION

Exfoliation treatments are gaining popularity and are available in many forms. Exfoliation is the controlled removal of dead skin cells and other debris from the skins surface in order to give it a healthier sheen. It is understood that as we age the sloughing off of old skin cells is delayed. With treatments that utilize exfoliation, we can aid the sloughing process to expose younger, fresher, healthier looking skin. Exfoliation can range from treatments consisting of enzymes, scrubs, or brushing techniques, to alpha or beta hydroxy acids. Oftentimes, exfoliation treatments are done in conjunction with bath treatments or hydrotherapy. The popularity of water treatments and the use of baths have resurfaced and are fast becoming a highly requested spa treatment. Baths can be used in a relaxing or therapeutic manner and can include a wide variety of additives and different temperature ranges. Both exfoliation and bath treatments complement each other and can be used together or alone in any spa.

■ EXFOLIATING TREATMENTS

Exfoliating treatments are effective for exfoliating the outermost skin cells, revealing a fresh and glowing skin tone. They are available in the form of scrubs, hydroxy acids, and masks. They have become very popular in spas. Exfoliating treatments can be used individually or in preparation for many other body treatments.

Sea Salts or Salt Glow

A **sea scrub** or **salt glow** utilizes minerals from the seas, in particular, the Dead Sea, to exfoliate and replenish the skin. The Dead Sea, despite its name, is the most mineral rich body of water in the world. Mineral extraction from the Dead Sea for medical and aesthetic use has become a cottage industry. One of the aesthetic uses is to make sea salt scrubs. Sea salt scrubs are one of the most popular body treatments at spas and can be performed with or without a wet room. It stimulates the circulation, exfoliates the outermost skin cells, moisturizes the skin, and reveals a fresh and glowing skin tone. Because the salt or sea scrub is usually combined with aromatic oil, it hydrates the skin. (See Figure 7–1.) The traditional method of removal of this treatment is with a shower or warm towels.

The treatment may be followed with the application of body lotion or other treatments such as seaweed or algae, which are complemented by the exfoliation benefits this treatment provides. A salt glow can also be combined with a massage. It is recommended to get the salt glow first

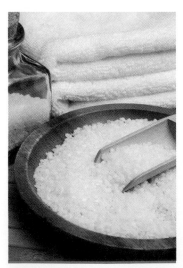

Figure 7–1 Salt scrubs are a popular treatment in the spa today

Salt Glow Recipe:

1. Combine two parts of salt (sea salt or pickling salt) to one part oil of grape seed or almond oil.
2. Add one to two teaspoons of essential oil for every two cups of scrub. (Good choices include lavender, spearmint, and eucalyptus.
3. Mix well. For best results, store in a cool area.

   The scrub will remove dead skin cells, and the essential oils will draw out toxins for up to two hours following the treatment.[1]

because it is stimulating, whereas the massage is soothing. Some spas have signature treatments that combine both services.

Muds and Clays

The formation of **muds** and clays begins with fine sediments eroded from rocks and carried away by water along with decaying organic material and other natural sediments. The mud's color, odor, and other special properties and characteristics are dependant upon its composition and place of origin. The spa industry is interested in the muds thermal, mechanical, and chemical therapeutic properties.[2]

Muds and clays have been used for hundreds of years for many cosmetic and therapeutic effects. The specific therapeutic effects will be dependant upon the specific clay's point of origin, as chemical compositions will vary accordingly. (See Figure 7–2.) As an aesthetician, you should be aware of the muds and clays you use, particularly their points of origin, and the specific therapeutic effects.

muds

along with clays begin with the erosion of rocks, usually carried away by flowing water and deposits along with decaying organic material and sediments at riversides or at the bottom of seas and lakes; used in spa treatments to refine the skin

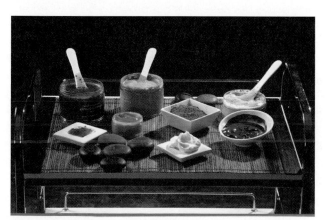

Figure 7–2 Muds and clays have been used for hundreds of years for many cosmetic and therapeutic effects

Suggested Steps of a Dead Sea or Salt Glow Scrub Procedure

1. Prepare the treatment table with protective covering (i.e., sheet, plastic protector sheet, and a top sheet or towel). Place the scrub in a bowl and prepare for application.

2. Instruct the client to get onto the treatment table just below the top sheet or towel while you step outside the room.

3. Begin application at the feet and work up the entire body in an upward and gentle circular motion using the hands, exfoliating gloves, or a loofah mitt. Be careful to avoid any scratched or wounded areas. A dry brushing technique can also be used, but remember to consider the client's skin type when choosing the level of exfoliation.

4. First apply the mixture to the legs and buttocks area. Gently raise the knees. Apply the mixture to the feet and the front and back of the legs, before proceeding to the stomach, chest, and arms. Pay special attention to drier areas, such as the heels of the feet and the elbows, if necessary.

5. Instruct the client to cross his/her arms to hold the modesty towel in place and assist him/her into a sitting position. Apply the mixture with your hands to the back and shoulders. Assist the client back into the supine position.

6. Using the same steps as above, remove the product thoroughly with warm, moist towels (redraping as each area is addressed) or assist the client into the shower. If your client is not showering, roll or fold away the plastic protector sheet to provide a clean surface for him/her to lie on. It is important to remove all traces of the scrub because it will not prove relaxing when applying any after products or continuing with other treatments. Finish with a dry towel rub.

7. If desired, apply body lotion or massage cream, using light effleurage movements.

8. Inform the client of any specific posttreatment instructions.

Applications of these masks are made specific to the areas of concern, such as face, abdomen, or legs. (See Figure 7–3.) They are rich in herbal minerals and are among the most valuable skin therapy treatments for rehydration, detoxification, and nourishment. A good example is clay and its astringent effects upon the skin; as it dries it contracts, yielding firmness and eliminating dead skin cells.

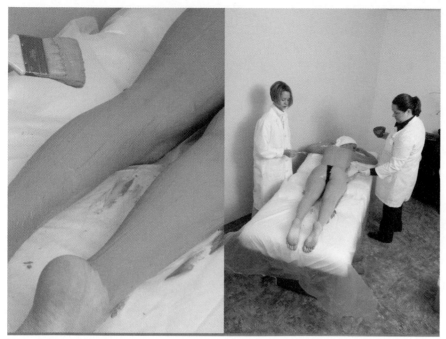

Figure 7–3 Applications of clay or mud masks are made specific to the areas of concern, such as face, abdomen, or legs

By using the body's own internal heat to assist in the purification process during the treatment, muds and clays have an added thermal component. Because they act as a drying agent, it is important to avoid overuse, as some muds and clays will cause excessive drying of the skin. It is advisable to moisten and replenish the skin to restore any moisture loss after these treatments.

Mud baths are popular in spas today. As with masks, the type of mud bath may be used to address the client's specific issues, but all rely on the same premise of the mud's own natural medium of water, herbs, and minerals.

Mud used for these treatments should always be of the highest quality. It should also be free of harmful components, such as pesticides and bacteria, and should contain only a moderate amount of minerals. One of the more popular modalities, **ayurveda**, works on the principles of combining mud with herbs.

ayurveda
an Indian word that is translated as the knowledge of how to live

Dead Sea Mud and Salts

As mentioned, the Dead Sea's black mud has been used for therapeutic purposes since ancient times. Its healing powers are mentioned in the Bible, and have been used by ancient royalty such as Cleopatra, the

Suggested Steps for a Hand Treatment

1. Massage an exfoliator onto moistened skin for a few minutes on each hand. (If the client wishes to address age spots, an enzyme, light glycolic peel, or microdermabrasion may be performed in place of the exfoliation.)
2. Rinse and dry well. (Hot moistened towels may be used for added relaxation to remove exfoliation grains.)
3. Mix a supple hand cream with a few drops of an antiaging or glycolic serum and apply to the hands.
4. Cover with the heated mitts or cotton gloves. Leave in place for 15 to 20 minutes.
5. Remove the gloves or mitts and massage in the residual product.

Suggested Steps for a Foot Treatment

1. Spread an exfoliator on moistened skin, massage for a few minutes. (Massage upwards toward the heart.) The lower leg area may also be treated.
2. Rinse with water. Pat gently to dry. (Hot moistened towels may be used for added relaxation.)
3. Spread a generous layer of nourishing foot cream onto the feet.
4. Apply a moisturizing or nourishing mask and leave to set for 15 minutes.
5. Rinse and dry thoroughly. (Hot moistened towels may be used for added relaxation.)

Complete treatment by applying a stimulating or refreshing foot cream combined with a stimulating foot massage.

Queen of Sheba, and King Herod the Great. Aristotle, the Greek philosopher, even wrote about the remarkable waters of the Dead Sea, which is located in Southeastern Asia at the Earth's lowest point (400 meters below sea level).

The Dead Sea has a 33 to 35 percent concentration of salts and minerals (compared to the ocean's 3 percent) and contains 21 minerals composed of a unique chemical composition of chloride, sodium, potassium, calcium, bicarbonate, sulfate, and magnesium. Of these 21 minerals, 12 are found in no other sea or ocean. Because of its high salt content and the density of solids in the water, the Dead Sea provides bathers with effort-free buoyancy.[3]

People visit the Dead Sea to benefit from the therapeutic powers of its water and mud and to seek treatment for dermatological and rheumatic disorders. The waters of the Dead Sea are believed to be ideal for treating eczema, psoriasis, acne, and several other skin ailments. It is believed that the therapeutic properties of the Dead Sea are primarily due to the unique balance and presence of key minerals, including magnesium, iodine, sulfur, potassium, and bromide.

A series of clinical research projects have been carried out in other countries, including Israel, examining the use of the Dead Sea's harvested salts in therapeutic baths. The data compiled by the studies demonstrated a substantial improvement in both skin and rheumatory conditions, yielding more pronounced improvements with individuals with greater physical limitations and conditions.

The Dead Sea salts that are commercially used in spas today are obtained by a method of crystallization and fractional evaporation. This process retains mineral elements and enriches the therapeutically valuable magnesium and potassium salts.[4]

Fango Mud

Fango, the Italian word for "mud," has been providing therapeutic efficacy since ancient Roman time. Fango mud is sometimes made of pure volcanic ash. (See Figure 7–4.) The compound is mixed with thermal water that is rich in salt, bromine, and iodine, and a number of other organic components, such as algae and protozoa. It is often fortified with salicyl (aspirin) for maximum therapeutic effect. Ensuring that fango mud is mature is one of the most important aspects of **fangotherapy**.

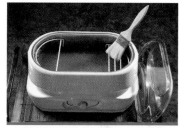

Figure 7–4 "Fango" is the Italian word for mud. This is an example of parafango.

Fango mud therapy is mostly used in thermal centers or "thermae." These centers have a long history of being a centerpiece in Italian and many European cultures. The word "thermae" originates from the Greek word meaning warm, and was used to describe an urban structure very popular in ancient Rome: public baths of huge proportions with great pools of different temperatures. These thermae were usually donated by an emperor or a govenor. The infamous Italian Emperor Caracalla (A.D. 188–217) extended Roman citizenship to all freemen in the empire with the goal of raising enough taxes for his famous projects including Thermae Caracalla. Thermae Caracalla, located in Italy, in its day could host more than 1,600 guests and was characterized by extraordinary splendor. It contained several bathing options for the guests, including underground vaulted facilities for servicing the calidarium (hot baths) and tepidarium (lukewarm baths).

The Roman thermae were also centers for the practice of medical and cosmetic treatments, sports, physical exercise, and musical entertainment

fango
the Italian word for "mud"; a gray-brown clay-like compound is mixed with thermal water that is rich in salt, bromine, iodine, and a number of other organic components, such as algae and protozoa

fangotherapy
the use of fango mud

and as such became places for socialization, amusement, and therapy. In Italy after the medieval period, a movement by popes and the culture of the Renaissance was to restore many of the thermae and initiate further searches for new sources of thermal waters.

The mineral rich springs supplying the thermal water are used for baths, mud therapy, inhalation, and rehabilitation procedures. Each source of thermal water is supplied by different springs with different characteristics and properties. In Italy (as well as many European countries that value these characteristics and healing properties), the sources are constantly tested and monitored by the Italian Ministry of Health. A typical thermal spring is 149° Fahrenheit, and contains sodium, chloride, bicarbonate, sulfate, calcium, magnesium, bromine, and iodine ions. There is also high-to-low water radioactivity (depending on the well) within the therapeutic range, due to dissolved radon.

Italy is still a popular spot for retreats to thermal spas and thermal centers. Medical hydrology and thermal medicine are taught in seven university medical schools in Italy, as part of the predoctoral medical disciplines, and as postgraduate and specialization courses. The Italian National Health System officially recognizes the efficacy and safety of the thermal water and mud therapies. Many Italian citizens are reimbursed for therapies received at thermal centers.

In most thermal spas, clays of different origins (volcanic, pale marine, moraine) are selected according to their structure, permeability, and aggregation state. Most clay is basically argil: a conglomeration of crystalline minerals (silicates and hydrates of colloidal aluminum). Thermal water originates through a complex process, deep within the earth. Water travels in high flow systems through complex channels of faults in the earth (fissures of the earth's crust). The water becomes superheated, attributing to gradual mineralization, with the end product being extremely rich in minerals. In thermal spas, the waters from the mineral rich springs supplying the thermal water are used for baths, mud therapy, inhalation, and rehabilitation procedures. The mud is matured for six months to one year in huge outdoor pools and during this time is continuously immersed in running thermal water from the selected source.

To produce true fango mud, the mud must undergo a somewhat complex, scientific maturation process that usually includes maintaining the mud at a constant temperature and passing it through a series of holding areas while in direct contact with thermal water, sunlight, and air.

The mud undergoes radical transformations in its physical and chemical characteristics, forming new molecular ties with the minerals (transmineralization). The temperature of the water allows the mud to be enriched with mineral salts and nonmineral elements in a way that is not possible with water at lower temperatures. Most importantly, it also becomes enriched with organic compounds, deriving from the particular microflora (bacteria, algae, protozoa, etc.), microfauna, humus, and humus-mineral compounds of the maturation pools. During this maturation process, the mud is gradually enriched with organic substances such as mineral salts and a particular form of surface algae, which thrives in environments of rich mineral content and very high temperatures. Maturation of the fango mud ensures its efficacy is strengthened by its ability to give off heat. The heating component found with fango leads to several physiological effects, including detoxification, anti-inflammatory effects, analgesia, muscle relaxation, and revitalization.

When it comes to mud therapy, an excellent model to follow is that of the European spas, where fangotherapy is taken seriously. Most have an on-site physician who develops a treatment protocol specifying the temperature of the mud, which body parts will receive the treatments, and how long the treatment will last. The medical mud treatment cycle typically consists of 12 mud treatments (15 minutes each, one per day), possibly interrupted for one day after days four and eight. Each mud treatment, in the typical cycle, is followed by a 15 minute thermal water shower or immersion in a thermal ionized bath at an optimal temperature of 100° Fahrenheit, for 10 minutes. The thermal bath helps to relax the muscles and dilate the blood vessels, stimulating circulation (patients with heart or blood vessel conditions ought to consult a physician prior to any treatment). The next step is a 30 minute relaxation phase of sweating and cooling down while wrapped in blankets or a hooded robe. The final step may include a full-body stimulating massage to obtain a toning effect.[5]

Because certain medicinal properties of the medical grade mud are retained for only 1 to 2 days outside the thermal source, the mud can be harvested for cosmetic purposes and taken out of the environment that maintains the medicinal properties. Properties valued at the cosmetic level are retained throughout and remain beneficial at the cosmetic level. A spa will use commercially packaged cosmetic grade muds for body and facial treatments. Commercially manufactured, nonmatured mud may be composed of components such as mineral rich volcanic ash and can be used in a mud bath, as a component of a wrap, or in conjunction with a paraffin treatment. When performing fango body wraps, the body is dry brushed, painted with fango mud, and wrapped in warm blankets. This treatment soothes tired, sore muscles and cleanses the skin. The warming fango mud helps to replenish skin cells and relax joints and muscles.[6]

Peat Therapy and Moor Mud

Peat therapy in health care and balneology has dated back to early Celtic and Roman baths. Modern peat therapy spas include Europe, Czech

peat therapy
uses peat mud and peat suspension baths in balneotherapy and poultices

moor mud
a natural peat preparation, rich in organic matter, proteins, vitamins, and trace minerals, is known for penetrating the skin, influencing enzymatic and hormone activity

fruit scrubs
usually refer to a mixture of an exfoliating granule and an alpha hydroxy acid used as an exfoliation product and work by dissolving the cellular cement that holds dead skin cells together, revealing a smoother, more even skin tone and promoting an increased cellular turnover

alpha hydroxy acids
mild organic acids used in cosmeceutical products. AHAs "unglue" cells in the epidermis, allowing keratinocytes to be shed at the stratum granulosum, providing skin with a healthier texture

glycolic acid
alpha hydroxy acid derived from sugar cane; it has a small molecular size that allows for easier penetration into the skin

malic acid
an AHA derived from apples

citric acid
an AHA derived from citrus fruit (e.g., oranges and grapefruit)

lactic acid
an AHA derived from milk

Republic, Germany, and Austria. Peat is found in peat lands or mires, otherwise known as wetland ecosystems, and its quality is dependant on the bog from which it is harvested. The majority of the peat lands are found in the Northern Hemisphere's temperate cold belt, with the remaining 10 percent hidden under foliage in the subtropics and tropics. The peat is produced as a heterogeneous mixture of more than a thousand organic materials accumulating at a rate higher than decomposition. The humus (decomposing plant material) and by-products of the accumulating matter thrive in a wet, oxygen poor environment while optimal temperatures promote plant growth and inhibiting the overabundance of decomposing organisms.[7]

Moor mud, a natural peat preparation, rich in organic matter, proteins, vitamins, and trace minerals, is known for penetrating the skin, influencing enzymatic and hormone activity. Common peloids, such as Dead Sea mud, volcanic mud, and clay muds, which are used in the beauty industry, are almost entirely composed of inorganic substances, some of which have molecular structures that are too large to penetrate the skin.

Moor mud is noted for its use as an effective natural product for the treatment of arthritis, chronic skin conditions, and stomach ailments. It is also an excellent choice for a general detoxification program. Common uses for moor mud include baths, wraps, and moor mud packs.

Moor mud packs look like giant tea bags, with one side porous to allow the contents of the pack to penetrate into the skin. The other side is composed of a nonporous material, which is heated by the aid of a heat-carrier-gel pack to heat the moor mud to an optimal temperature of 140° Fahrenheit.[8]

Moor mud helps to eliminate aches and discomfort from the body while soothing the skin. This treatment begins with a mud exfoliation followed by a moor mud wrap. The body is cocooned for 20 minutes while a gentle massage is given to the head to encourage relaxation. After the wrap, the body is rinsed using a vichy shower and tenderly dried. An application of moor body crème concludes the service, with the client emerging from the cocoon feeling beautiful and refreshed.

Fruit Scrubs

Fruit scrubs usually refer to a mixture of an exfoliating granule and an alpha hydroxy acid used as an exfoliation product. (See Figure 7–5.) **Alpha hydroxy acids** are acids derived from the sugars in particular plants. These acids work by dissolving the cellular cement that holds dead skin cells together, revealing a smoother, more even skin tone and promoting an increased cellular turnover. Some examples include **glycolic acid**, **malic acid**, **citric acid**, and **lactic acid**. (See Table 7–1.)

Suggested Steps for a Moor Mud Pack Treatment

1. Cover up the untreated area to maintain body heat.
2. Large packs are usually placed on the treatment table. Have the client lay directly on the packs. The packs feel slightly damp and are very soothing as the heat builds up. As the pores open from the increasing heat, toxins and bacteria are released from the skin's cells and are absorbed by the pack.
3. Process the client for about 30 minutes.
4. Wipe the client with a warm moist towel to remove any residue.

This is a relatively mess-free, relaxing, and therapeutic treatment any client would enjoy.[9]

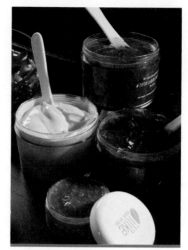

Figure 7–5 Fruit scrubs usually refer to a mixture of an exfoliating granule and an alpha hydroxy acid used as an exfoliation product

▪ PARAFFIN

Paraffin treatments, which provide many benefits to the client, have gained in popularity at spas. They are easy to add to an existing menu as the start-up fees are minimal. It is also an easy procedure to learn.

Originally, warm paraffin treatments were prescribed for pain relief and were used only by the medical community to soothe aches and pains due to arthritis, joint stiffness, sport injury, or overuse. Over time, the treatment has moved into spas where the advantage is taken of the warm wax to stimulate circulation and facilitate the penetration of rich creams or serums and ampoules.

Paraffin treatments are ideal for dry and dehydrated skin. Paraffin is also used in the form of heated packs.

Paraffin is an alkaline wax with many uses from fuel (kerosene) to aesthetic purposes.

Table 7–1	Fruits Used for Scrubs
Fruits	**Essential Oils**
Apricot	Lavender
Mandarin Orange	Sunflower Seeds
Lemon	Carrot Seeds
Banana	Olive
Papaya	
Watermelon	
Pineapple	

Suggested Steps for a Moor Mud Body Treatment

1. Prepare the treatment table with a protective covering (i.e., sheet, plastic protector sheet, wool blanket, cellophane sheet or space blanket, and a top sheet or towel). Place the moor mud in a bowl and prepare for application. Store the mud in the hot towel cabbie until it is needed.

2. Instruct the client to get onto the treatment table just below the top sheet or towel while you step outside of the room. When you return and prior to the application of the mud, perform an exfoliating pretreatment of dry brushing with a natural bristle body brush using the following procedure:

    a. Brush following the natural direction of lymphatic glands to encourage their drainage in the most effective method. Begin brushing upward from the ankles, up the legs, and toward the heart, using six to eight long strokes on each area of the body.

    b. To easily reach the back of the legs, gently raise the knees and work toward the buttocks.

    c. When brushing the abdominal area, brush down the abdomen using a clockwise motion, following the action of the intestines, toward the lymph nodes in the groin area.

    d. Brush the décolleté, avoiding the breasts, in upward strokes toward the lymph nodes in the neck.

    e. The arms, shoulders, and back should be brushed toward the nodes in the axilla area. To reach the back and shoulder area, instruct the client to cross his/her arms to hold the modesty towel in place and assist him/her into a sitting position.

3. Apply the moor mud with the client still sitting in the upright position. Apply the mixture with hands or an oversized brush to the back and shoulders.

4. Next assist the client back to the supine position and begin to apply the mixture to the legs and buttocks area, draping to prevent heat loss as you proceed.

5. Gently raise the knees and apply the mixture to the feet and front and back of the legs before proceeding to the stomach, chest, and arms.

6. Begin wrapping the client with plastic wrap and a space blanket while removing the top sheet or towel so that the cellophane is touching the client's skin directly.

7. Next fold up the layers or blankets onto the client. Use a towel around the neck area to prevent heat loss.

8. Process for the desired time, which is usually 25 minutes. Place a cool cloth on the client's head, if desired, during the processing time.

9. Fold down the plastic sheet and blankets. Remove product thoroughly with warm moist towels, redraping as each area is addressed, or assist the client into the shower.

10. Remove all soiled linens so the client will be on a clean dry surface.

11. If preferred, apply body lotion or massage cream, using light effleurage movements.

12. Offer the client water to drink to rehydrate him/her. Inform him/her of any specific posttreatment instructions.[10]

Suggested Steps for a Fruit Scrubs Body Treatment

1. Prepare treatment table with protective covering (i.e., sheet, plastic protector sheet, wool blanket, and a top sheet or towel).

2. Instruct the client to get onto the treatment table just below the top sheet or towel while you step outside of the room.

3. When you return, prepare the body with a hydroxy acid cleansing gel or lotion, depending on the skin type. Use light **effleurage** movements over the entire body. Rinse with large wet sponges. For a more luxurious feel, use hot moist towels.

4. Spray appropriate hydroxy acid toner with the Lucas spray or desired applicator. Penetrate the toner until absorption is achieved, using light effleurage movements.

5. Apply the exfoliating fruit scrub by hand or with a brush, massaging in a circular motion. This is also an appropriate time to use a steamer. For a stand-alone steamer, move it up and down the body, focusing on the area being exfoliated. Rinse with large wet sponges. For a more luxurious feel, use hot moist towels. Remember to maintain proper draping, exposing only the area that is currently being worked on. (Because of the different manufacturers of scrubs, the hydroxy acid content may vary. Remember to follow the manufacturer's specific instructions for the processing time or the application procedure.)

6. As in Step 2, spray appropriate toner with the Lucas spray or desired applicator. Penetrate the toner until absorption is achieved, using light effleurage movements.

7. Apply a finishing cream to the body, using light effleurage movements. Some manufacturers also include a hydroxy acid cream during this step to get further benefits of exfoliation, but remember to consider your client's skin sensitivity levels when adjusting your protocols.

8. Help the client turn over, maintaining the appropriate draping protocols. Repeat these steps on the other side of the body.

effleurage
the massage movement using the palmar aspect of the hand or pads of the fingertips to produce a soothing effect

Parafango Packs

Parafango is a mixture of fango mud and paraffin. (See Figure 7–6.) It can be mixed to yield an extremely plastic mass that is easily molded to fit any part of the body. Parafango packs, if completely dehydrated, allow a greater heat exchange to take place. The heat transmission of these dehydrated packs is high and continual (as opposed to a mixture with higher

parafango
a mixture of fango mud and paraffin

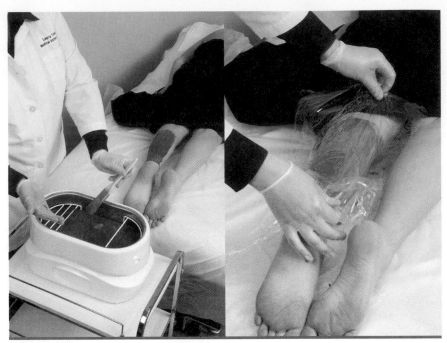

Figure 7–6 Application of a parafango pack

liquid content) and can be heated to higher temperatures. The packs are placed on different parts of the body. One pack can be used on an isolated body part or applied to several areas at once.

Application of Parafango Packs

Parafango packs create a mini-sauna environment that revitalizes the skin, relaxes the client, improves blood circulation, reduces muscular tension, and increases the elimination of toxins. They are administered in hot packs onto the desired site at approximately 100° Fahrenheit for 20 minutes. (See Figure 7–7.)

Paraffin in Everyday Use

When visiting a spa, clients are looking for a more luxurious atmosphere—one with all the extras. Paraffin treatments contribute to this atmosphere, as they are a great add-on service to any facial, manicure, pedicure, or body treatment.

Paraffin treatments are easy to learn and integrate. They require a minimal investment of a temperature regulated heater, paraffin, and service specific tools such as hand and foot cream, gauze (used to apply the paraffin), plastic protectors, and cotton mitts or booties (when integrated into a manicure or pedicure).

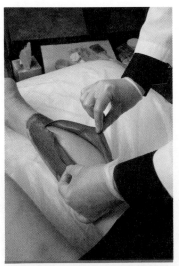

Figure 7–7 Removal of a parafango pack

To address hygiene concerns, it is recommended that gauze be dipped into the paraffin and then applied to the area versus dipping the client's hands or feet directly into the bath itself. Applications with brushes also pose a double-dipping hazard and are not recommended for this treatment.

BATHS

The history of public baths, which were found throughout Europe, can be traced back to ancient Rome when Roman men and women would try to visit the baths at least once every day. The baths were popular spots for men to gather to discuss business and important issues and were frequented for relaxation purposes as well. Some establishments would allow women to visit at specific times. The poor and children were not allowed.

Today, there are many historic sites to visit that still maintain these traditional public baths. Modified versions are gaining in popularity in larger spas as well. The spa industry is also taking advantage of the growing interest in relaxation by developing home bath treatments for clients to relax and enjoy in the privacy of their own homes.[11]

The Purpose of Baths

Baths rely on healing properties, based on thermal and mechanical factors. The bath works with the skin's touch receptors and the body's nervous system. The weightlessness of the body, the pressure of the water, and the temperature stimuli all invoke physiological reactions. A warm bath also encourages a state of relaxation by slowing the body down and easing muscle tension and stresses. A cold bath, on the other hand, is invigorating and increases activity. It is recommended to take a warm bath, followed by a short integrating cold shower.[12]

The Use of Aromatherapy in Baths

Certain aromatherapy essential oils are quite effective for creating soothing baths, relaxing muscles and easing joints, or for addressing skin conditions. Placing a few drops of lavender, soaking for 30 minutes in the tub while meditating, listening to tranquil music, or just relaxing has great stress relieving benefits. A bath can be prepared specific to your goal by adjusting the essential oil that is added to the water. Please remember that essential oils are very concentrated and must be used with caution. Always be aware of the contraindications of each essential oil.[13] This information can often be found on the packaging.

There are many types of baths, all encouraging a state of relaxation.

■ DIFFERENT TYPES OF BATHS

A bath can be custom designed for each client's specific needs. There are many options, with each treatment having its own unique therapeutic effects. Hot or cold water, a stand-alone treatment, or a combination of herbs, oils, or mud or seaweed powders may be used. Baths may include aromatherapy and herbs, powders, fangos, milk, and sea salts. (See Table 7–2.) Fango natrium baths consist of volcanic ash, which is noted for minerals and trace elements that target detoxification, exfoliation, and relaxation. Milk baths take advantage of the lactic acid to soften dry and dehydrated skin. Sea salt baths usually contain Dead Sea salts, which are valued for trace elements and minerals.[14]

Healing Baths

healing baths
water treatments to address skin conditions, joint, muscle, or stress related disorders

Healing baths often bring to mind several types of conditions that would benefit from such a treatment, including skin conditions, and joint, muscle, or stress related disorders. Fango salicyl baths combine fango mud with aspirin derivatives and are used in a series to assist in soothing aching muscles and inflamed joints and to detoxify the body. (See Figure 7–8.) Oatmeal baths are also known for their healing process. They are used to remedy chicken pox, poison ivy, oak and sumac reactions, dry

Table 7–2	**Different Baths and Their Purposes**
Healing Baths	Remedy for skin conditions, joint, muscle, or stress related disorders
Seaweed Baths	Relaxation and blood flow stimulation
Watsu	Relaxation and stress reduction
Hot Springs	Relaxation and relief from pain due to inflammation
Sitz Bath	Assistance for increasing the blood flow to the pelvis and abdominal regions
Hot Footbaths	Increase of blood flow in the legs
Cold Footbaths	Increase of blood flow in the legs
Arm Baths	Remedy for respiratory problems
Steam Bath	Increase of blood flow, increase of the heart rate, opening of the airways, and relaxation of the muscles

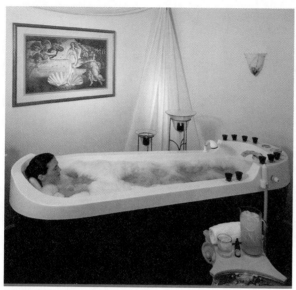

Figure 7–8 Relaxing in soothing water is a common spa treatment

skin, insect bites, eczema, diaper rash, sunburn, and shingles. Dead Sea salt baths are very popular in spas. Seawater has been used for thousands of years for its healing properties enriched with iodine, minerals, elements, and plankton. Mineral and hot spring waters also have many added health benefits.[15]

Seaweed Baths

Seaweed baths have gained in popularity in spas for relaxation purposes, for their ability to stimulate circulation and rid the body of toxins, and for their easy implementation. During a seaweed bath, micronized algae powder is added to temperature specific water. Because the algae have a strong odor, some manufacturers include an additional additive for the client's comfort. The benefits are gained from the algae's vitamins and minerals, such as copper, iron, potassium, zinc, and iodine, which can be absorbed by the skin. The overall benefit is detoxification, relaxation, and skin that looks and feels supple and smooth.[16]

Watsu

Watsu is the first form of aquatic bodywork that was developed in the 1980s by Harold Dull. Watsu, performed in warm water while the practitioner supports the floating client, combines the therapeutic benefits of warm water and the freedom of movement, joint mobilization, dance,

Thalassotherapy (Greek for "seawater") has been used as a healing tool for thousands of years.

seaweed baths
baths that use micronized algae powder added to the water

watsu
original aquatic spa treatment

stretching, massage, and shiatsu. It promotes a state of relaxation and stress reduction. It is considered by many to be one of the most profound developments in bodywork in our time. Watsu can be used as a stand-alone therapy or in conjunction with therapeutic work on land.[17]

Hot Springs, Thermal Springs, and Mineral Water

In the nineteenth century hot spring therapy became popular in the United States, attributing many health benefits to the use of therapeutic **geothermally** heated mineral waters with temperatures usually exceeding 175° Fahrenheit. The hot springs contain a multitude of chemical compounds and mineral properties, which are picked up underground as they travel to the surface. Today many hot springs are located in overnight spas and hotels and offer complete packages of complementary therapies.

There are two primary classifications of hot springs: primary and filtration. The difference is in the mineral and gas content of the water. While both are geothermally heated mineral water, **primary hot springs** water originates and is heated directly through volcanic activity, powered by magma chambers. Beginning at the surface as rainwater, **filtration hot springs** water travels through faults and fractures, exposed to gas and absorbing minerals as it is heated geothermally and returned to the surface.

There are several factors to consider when deciding on hot springs and their benefits. The first is the source, the second is the temperature, and the third is the mineral content. Many of the stimulating benefits of hot springs water are temperature dependant. It was found that soaking in optimally heated hot springs temporarily relieves pain due to inflammation.

The minerals dissolved in the water, such as sulfur, magnesium, calcium, potassium, sodium, and strontium, distinguish hot springs. This mineral composition provides different health benefits. Europeans have utilized bicarbonate waters for bathing to address hypertension and mild arteriosclerosis. Sodium assists with arthritic conditions and can stimulate lymphatic activity. Hot springs rich in sulfur address a wide variety of conditions, including ingestion for gastrointestinal or liver conditions, inhalation therapy for respiratory problems, and skin infections and inflammations.

Springs naturally rich in chlorides are found to be favorable for arthritis, rheumatic conditions, and numerous other conditions. Magnesium promotes healthy skin. Potassium also promotes healthy skin, as well as aids in reducing high blood pressure and the elimination of toxins.

---

geothermally
heated by the earth

primary hot springs
springs that are powered by magma chambers, miles under the earth's surface

filtration hot springs
geothermally heated mineral water that is fed by rain water that seeps into the earth through faults and fractures

In general, soaking in thermal and hot springs has a positive, sedative effect and relaxes muscles—something that everyone can benefit from in today's stressful world.[18]

Sitz Baths

A **sitz bath** is a form of hydrotherapy that assists with increasing the blood flow to the pelvis and abdominal regions. It is a shallow water bath, brewed with an herbal tea mixture such as comfrey, dried garlic and sea salt, uva ursi, and myrrh gum, which soaks only the lower body and thighs. It has proven to be very effective in easing pain after childbirth. Hot sitz baths, with temperatures around 110° Fahrenheit, last up to 40 minutes and are followed by a quick, cold shower or bath.

Hot sitz baths are used for hemorrhoids and abdominal cramps. Cold sitz baths are tubs that are filled with ice water, last only 30 to 60 seconds and are used for conditions that involve inflammation. Alternating hot and cold sitz baths is also useful for skin conditions such as eczema and psoriasis. With alternating baths, the hot bath lasts approximately three minutes and the cold, 30 to 60 seconds. The two are usually repeated three to four times each in one sitting.[19]

Footbaths

Footbaths come in two forms, hot and cold, with each one having its own indications. Cold footbaths are useful for circulatory problems, edema, low blood pressure, varicose veins, headaches, and other conditions. Hot footbaths are mostly used for cold feet and for relaxation.[20]

Hot Footbaths, Cold Footbaths, and Arm Baths

Rising temperature footbaths, or warm footbaths, can be performed daily and can last up to 15 minutes. (See Figure 7–9.) During these baths, the feet are immersed in a footbath that is filled with water at body temperature. Hot water is gradually added to give a final temperature of 103° to 104° Fahrenheit. Warm footbaths are contraindicative to individuals with edema, lymphostasis, or varicose veins.

Cold footbaths involve immersing the feet up to calf level in cold water. The bath is short in duration, lasting only until the water is no longer perceived as cold. This treatment is contraindicative to individuals with cold feet, very high blood pressure, and the loss of sensation or diabetes.

Arm baths can be cold, warm, or rising in temperature. Rising temperature arm baths are similar to rising temperature footbaths. They are indicated for respiratory problems such as bronchitis and asthma, as well

sitz bath
a form of hydrotherapy that assists with increasing the blood flow to the pelvis and abdominal regions

footbaths
water used to soak the feet

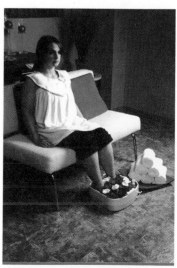

Figure 7–9 Footbaths are a pleasant way to begin a spa day

> Footbaths help alleviate minor foot pain and swelling, relaxing the client.

as circulatory problems, and are usually followed by a cold bath with a rest period of 30 minutes.

Cold arm baths are used for headaches and sleeplessness and should be avoided by individuals with circulatory and heart conditions. In a cold arm bath, a basin is filled with cold water just above the elbow.[21]

▪ STEAM BATH

A steam bath, which provides muscle relaxation and increased circulation due to the body's rise in temperature, is constructed from fiberglass, contains a seat for the client, and includes a hinged door with an opening at the top for the client's head to be exposed. The client sits on a seat inside the bath. The water is heated to a steam, which mixes with the air in the bath to produce a water vapor.

The temperature inside the cabinet is most comfortable at between 113° and 122° Fahrenheit lower than that of a sauna. The lower temperature is effective against causing the client to overheat, which is a major concern because the air in the steam bath is saturated with water vapor, inhibiting the skin from cooling through perspiration.[22]

▪ SAUNA

A sauna provides a dry heat treatment and is usually constructed of porous wood, such as pine, that allows the absorption of condensation and air inlets for circulation. The air is usually heated by an electric stove to between 155° and 230° Fahrenheit. Some saunas have stoves, which contain coals. Once the coals become hot, water is poured on top to produce a steam.

The sauna stimulates blood flow, increases the heart rate, opens the airways, and relaxes the muscles. Saunas are not indicated for those with acute rheumatoid arthritis, circulatory problems, or cancer. The maximum time spent in a sauna is around 15 to 20 minutes.[23]

Conclusion

There are many treatments available in spas today, most having a history dating back hundreds of years.[24] Many of Europe's spa therapies are re-emerging and becoming popular in the United States.[25] Exfoliation treatments and water therapy, including baths, are some of the more popular body treatments available. They can be luxurious and relaxing or they can be targeted for therapeutic benefits.

▶ ▷ ▷ TOP 10 TIPS TO TAKE TO THE CLINIC

1. Have your client conduct a thorough health screening.
2. Check for contraindications.
3. Be familiar with ingredients that typically are related to allergies.
4. Be familiar with treatments or ingredients that are hazardous to certain health conditions.
5. Never leave the client unattended.
6. Develop a protocol to address client allergies or reactions to promote safety.
7. Always prepare your room ahead of time.
8. Provide your client with water to drink to prevent dehydration.
9. Provide your client with take-home instructions to maximize the treatment benefits.
10. Offer home-care products to complement the treatments.

CHAPTER QUESTIONS

1. What is an exfoliating treatment?
2. What is the benefit of using a salt glow?
3. What is the benefit of a mud mask?
4. What is moor mud and where can it be found?
5. What is fango therapy?
6. Provide an example of a fruit scrub.
7. What is the purpose of paraffin treatments?
8. Describe the uses of parafango packs.
9. What are the benefits of parafango packs?
10. Name some everyday spa uses of paraffin.
11. Name two types of baths and their benefits.
12. What is the difference between a sauna and a steam bath?

CHAPTER REFERENCES

1. Worwood, V. (2001). *Aromatherapy for Beauty Therapist*. Clifton Park, NY: Thompson Delmar Learning.
2. http://www.centerchem.com

3. http://www.psoriasis.org
4. http://www.chemistrystore.com
5. http://www.teletour.it
6. http://www.teletour.it
7. http://www.peatsociety.org
8. Bergel, R., & Leavy, H. (2003). *The Spa Encyclopedia*. Clifton Park, NY: Thompson Delmar Learning.
9. http://www.templespa.ie
10. Nordmann, L. (2002). *Professional Beauty Therapy, The Official Guide to Level 3*. Clifton Park, NY: Thompson Delmar Learning.
11. Bergel, R., & Leavy, H. (2003). *The Spa Encyclopedia*. Clifton Park, NY: Thompson Delmar Learning.
12. Bergel, R., & Leavy, H. (2003). *The Spa Encyclopedia*. Clifton Park, NY: Thompson Delmar Learning.
13. Bergel, R., & Leavy, H. (2003). *The Spa Encyclopedia*. Clifton Park, NY: Thompson Delmar Learning.
14. Worwood, V. (2001). *Aromatherapy for Beauty Therapist*. Clifton Park, NY: Thompson Delmar Learning.
15. Bergel, R., & Leavy, H. (2003). *The Spa Encyclopedia*. Clifton Park, NY: Thompson Delmar Learning.
16. Bergel, R., & Leavy, H. (2003). *The Spa Encyclopedia*. Clifton Park, NY: Thompson Delmar Learning.
17. Bergel, R., & Leavy, H. (2003). *The Spa Encyclopedia*. Clifton Park, NY: Thompson Delmar Learning.
18. http://www.watsu.org.nz/
19. http://www.eytonsearth.org
20. Bergel, R., & Leavy, H. (2003). *The Spa Encyclopedia*. Clifton Park, NY: Thompson Delmar Learning.
21. Bergel, R., & Leavy, H. (2003). *The Spa Encyclopedia*. Clifton Park, NY: Thompson Delmar Learning.
22. Nordmann, L. (2002). *Professional Beauty Therapy, The Official Guide to Level 3*. Clifton Park, NY: Thompson Delmar Learning.
23. Nordmann, L. (2002). *Professional Beauty Therapy, The Official Guide to Level 3*. Clifton Park, NY: Thompson Delmar Learning.
24. http://www.eytonsearth.org
25. http://palimpsest.stanford.edu

Facials and Advanced Facial Treatments

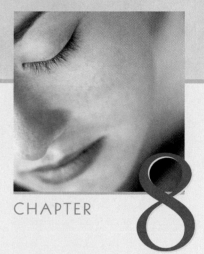

CHAPTER 8

LEARNING OBJECTIVES

After completing this chapter, you should be able to:

1. Discuss facials offered in the spa.

2. Discuss the use of aromatherapy with facials.

3. Discuss the steps for a facial and the common products used in facials.

4. Discuss facials using advanced technology or advanced product ingredients.

facials
treatments that cleanse, tone, purify, and stimulate or calm the skin

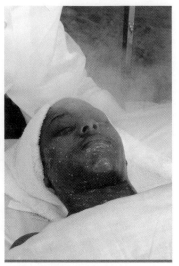

Figure 8–1 Facials are one of the most requested treatments at spas

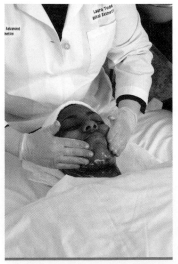

Figure 8–2 An aesthetician must master the basics of a facial by practicing the step-by-step movements in sequence

INTRODUCTION

Facials are one of the most requested treatments at spas, if not the single most requested treatment. Aside from being effective and noninvasive, they are beneficial in balancing, restoring, and nourishing the skin and relaxing the client. Today there exist a variety of facials that are desired by clients. (See Figure 8–1.) Many spas choose to offer facials that focus on a natural or machine-free approach. Other spas and clinics provide facials using machines or advanced technologies. The choice of which approach a clinician decides to take is based on personal preference. Many practitioners prefer the human touch, which is provided when performing manual or machine-free facials. At the other end of the spectrum is the practice of integrating machines into the facial with the premise that they may provide a more effective outcome. The outcomes achieved are not substantially different when discussing basic modalities such as steam towels versus a steamer or manual exfoliation versus machine-aided brushes. The margin begins to widen in the effectiveness achieved when discussing electrical modalities such as galvanic current including iontophoresis for product penetration versus a massage targeted to penetrate products. Without a doubt, the results are more effective with electrical modalities. Ultrasound is even more effective and has proven to be a popular choice with clinical based skin care practitioners.

FACILS

All basic facial treatments share several commonalities including cleansing, toning, exfoliating, massaging, and mask treatments. (See Figure 8–2.) Basic facials provide benefits such as general relaxation, exfoliation, deep cleansing, stimulating circulation and lymphatic drainage, and corrective properties. With all of the facial options that are available, it is not easy to determine which ones are the best. However, aestheticians should remember that there are two important things that guarantee their success:

- the ability to analyze the skin to determine the correct treatment
- the realization that expensive equipment is not needed to deliver effective results

When it comes to facials, an aesthetician's hands are one of the most powerful tools of the trade. One of the first things that every student learns in aesthetician school is the basic massage movements and manipulations, all performed by hand. It takes students several months to master the flow and appropriate pressure and touch. In addition, there are a wide variety of resources available today that can help deliver the desired results.

Organic Products

Because of the surge in the health and wellness industry, there has been an increase in the interest in organic products. Organic facial products usually contain all botanical ingredients, they are organically grown, hand-picked, and hand-harvested on either the manufacturer's own farm or by long term organic farmer partners, or they grow wild and are collected by the manufacturer in the woods and fields of rural areas. The organic ingredients are cold processed (no hydrogenation, no cooking) on the day of the harvest (the harvesting is done in small batches) into pulp format, and these pulps are usually stored in small batches such as five liter (five quart) jars under controlled circumstances to provide a fresh base for the products. The components used in the products are collected during the peak of the harvest season, and different herbs are usually collected at different times throughout the year. Because some of the products, such as the pulps, can be harvested only during peak season it is important to process them to provide ingredients that will last until the next harvest season.

Key factors in making organic products:

1. The formulas—The recipes for every product of the line are created and owned by the company. These are kept as secrets; most recipes are passed down generation to generation.
2. The manufacturing process—The work is done by hand; no mass production and special techniques are used to formulate the products.
3. The ingredients—It is very important that the herbal ingredients are grown in an environment that produces high quality components. The climate must be perfect for agriculture, and the soil must be extremely rich in minerals. Under proper soil conditions, the farmers will not need to use fertilizers, even if they are not organic farmers, because of the extremely rich soil providing superior amounts of necessary nutrients to the herbs, fruits, and vegetables:

   - vitamins
   - bioflavonoids
   - antioxidants
   - phytoestrogens
   - carotenoids and other pigments
   - bitter substances
   - fruit acids
   - glucose

- mineral salts
- trace elements
- many other important ingredients that nature can give us

Organic products can be very beneficial for clients and are very active with all natural ingredients and components. There is definitely a trend and a niche for these products in the marketplace.

Common Ingredients Used in Facials

There are certain common ingredients that are used in facials. Among those ingredients are alpha hydroxy acids, alpha lipoic acids, bentonite, green tea, and many others. The most commonly used ingredients are described below. (See Figure 8–3.)

Alpha Hydroxy Acid (AHA): This organic acid, taken from fruit acids, is used in antiaging skin care products to encourage moisture restoration and exfoliation and helps other ingredients to penetrate through the skin more effectively. It must be used in combination with sunscreen.

Alpha Lipoic Acid: This has anti-inflammatory benefits, plus it is water and fat soluble to protect skin cells.

Bentonite: This mineral-rich clay is used in facial masks for its oil-absorbing and deep-cleansing properties.

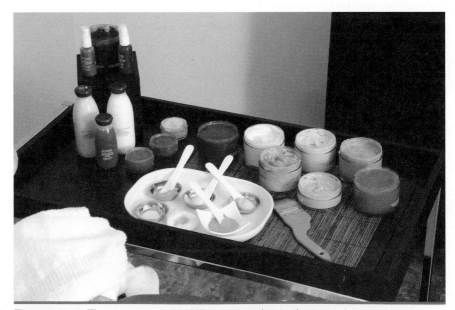

Figure 8–3 There are many different products that can be used to customize a facial

Benzoyl Peroxide: This powerful antibacterial agent helps kill acne by drying P. acnes bacteria on the skin.

Beta Hydroxy Acid: This oil soluble organic acid (salicylic acid) is used in exfoliators and acne treatments.

Collagen: The main epidermal protein, this is added to topical creams for its moisturizing benefits. (Collagen applied to the skin will not penetrate to produce collagen; it only moisturizes the skin.)

Elastin: A protein in the dermis, this is added for its moisturizing effects. (Elastin applied to the skin will not penetrate to produce elastin; it only moisturizes the skin.)

Enzymes: These are plant-based products that are used to digest the unwanted protein to reveal healthier skin.

Grape Seed Extract: This is a botanical extract known to increase the effectiveness of vitamin C by acting as a vehicle and a restorer of oxidized vitamin C.

Green Tea Extract: This derivative from decaffeinated green tea contains "catechins," which are effective antioxidants known to help prevent cancer.

Hyaluronic Acid: This is also known as "cyclic acid" and is a powerful moisturizing agent.

Hydroquinone: This is a skin lightening agent.

Kaolin: Also called china clay, this fine clay is white in color. Kaolin is often used in facial masks and powders that absorb oil.

Lactic Acid: This is used in chemical peels to hydrate, moisturize, and strip away dry, flaky skin cells.

Retinol: This is a fat soluble vitamin A. Retinol is crucial for good vision and healthy skin and is commonly used in antiaging preparations.

Salicylic Acid: This is a mild beta hydroxy acid that is used as a safe exfoliator in chemical peels for oilier skin types.

Sulfur: This essential mineral module of vitamin B kills bacteria causing acne and is found in many masks.

Titanium Dioxide: A chemical substance used in sunscreen products that blocks both UVA and UVB sun rays.

Vitamin A: This is a fat soluble vitamin that keeps skin hydrated. Vitamin A is used in skin care products because it improves aging skin and firms skin texture. It can also dry out acne and must be used in conjunction with sunscreens.

Vitamin C: This water soluble vitamin is used in cosmetic creams as well as in topical and oral medicines to boost collagen synthesis.

Vitamin D: This is a fat soluble vitamin that is used in some prescription medicines to treat psoriasis.

Vitamin E: This is an oil soluble antioxidant that is used to speed healing as well as to soften skin.

Witch Hazel: This is an effective astringent extracted from the leaves and bark of the Hamamelis Virginnia plant. It has botanical properties, helps improve acne, awakens puffy eyes, and reduces excess oil on the skin. This should be avoided on clients with rosacea.

Aromatherapy and Facials

Incorporating aromatherapy into a facial regime can be beneficial in several ways. Applying diluted oils to the skin directly benefits the client, and the aroma is relaxing for both the client and the practitioner. Because aromatherapy works on the olfactory nerves, located within the nasal cavity, both the client and the practitioner can receive the benefits during the treatment. (See Table 8–1.) Aromatherapy can be used in facials at many junctures. Essential oils can be added to towels, be included in

Table 8–1   Common Essential Oils and Their Uses
Bergamot: relaxes and refreshes, provides skin care, uplifts
Clary Sage: balances hormones, relieves muscle aches, relaxes
Eucalyptus: relieves muscle tension, alleviates respiratory problems, boosts the immune system
Frankincense: controls tension, helps to focus the mind, provides skin care
Geranium: balances hormones in women, provides skin care, relaxes
Neroli: relaxes and soothes, uplifts, provides skin care
Lavender: provides skin care, relaxes, and heals wounds
Lemon: relaxes, uplifts, heals wounds
Peppermint: relieves headaches, eases digestive disorders, relieves muscle aches
Tea Tree: provides antifungal treatment, strengthens immune system, provides skin care
Roman Chamomile: relaxes; heals wounds; relieves anxiety, muscle aches, and tension
Rosemary: strengthens immune system, relieves muscle aches, stimulates
Ylang Ylang: relaxes, relieves muscle tension[1]

the product itself, or be used in a room in the form of a spray. Essential oils work through aroma, and many work through the skin as well. Two common oils used in facials are lavender and rose. Lavender is undoubtedly the most versatile and useful of oils. It relaxes, soothes, restores, and balances the body and mind, calming or stimulating according to the body's needs. Rose oil has a wonderful scent and is an excellent choice for tired skin. It is frequently used for cleansing, toning, moisturizing, and nourishing the skin. Many manufacturers of product lines include aromatherapy of some sort in their formulations or treatment protocols. It is important to remember that essential oils must be diluted according to the manufacturer's direction and many oils can have contraindications. To master aromatherapy, it is advisable to take an entire class to learn all of the important points prior to using in protocols.

Steps to a Facial

There are seven basic steps to a facial:[2] A typical facial begins with light cleansing, which removes makeup and prepares the skin for the second step, the analysis. The third step provides deeper cleansing, exfoliation, and extractions, followed by the fourth step, the treat and correct phase. The facial then proceeds to wind down with a relaxing massage for step five, followed by a corrective mask for step six, and then finishes with the completion phase of a moisturizer or a specialty cream and sun protection. Basic facials used in the United States differ slightly from European facials. European facials typically are longer in length (90 to 120 minutes), focus more on specialty massage for product penetration or condition correction (lymphatic drainage or acupressure massage). European facials and American based facials typically incorporate the same steps but the steps may be followed in a different sequence. [See "Suggested Steps for a European Facial (Manual Facial)."]

Critical thinking skills, defined as using cognitive skills or strategies that increase the probability of a desired outcome, must be used when performing facials. Because every client is different, the facial should be customized to meet his or her specific needs. (See Table 8–2.) In aesthetician school you are given the basic tools such as knowledge of product ingredients and treatment protocols to apply and formulate each treatment to be specific to the client's needs. Each time your client returns you may have to adjust your protocol to target his or her specific goals. Aestheticians who get in a mind-set of "one size fits all" is really not providing their clients with the treatments they deserve. It is the ability to apply these skills appropriately to individual clients that sets a good aesthetician apart from his or her colleagues. It also ensures optimal outcomes and results. We have previously established that there are some basic components to a facial, and it is the manipulation of these steps to

Oxygen facials have become very popular over the past several years. There is quite a debate as to the efficacy of this treatment. Does it work? Does it provide true scientific results? The reality is that oxygen is carried through the bloodstream and nourishes the dermis from the blood supply. There is no evidence that the oxygen sprayed on the skin during a facial has any long term benefit to the skin.

Table 8–2	Different Facials and Their Benefits

Acne and Problem Skin Facial: To deep cleanse pores and balance oil production, extraction of comedones

AHA, BHA or Enzyme Facial: To improve the texture of the skin by removing excess buildup of cells

Antiaging Firming Facial: To firm the skin, stimulate metabolism, and add antioxidant ingredients

Deep Cleansing Facial: To thoroughly cleanse, extract comedones, and hydrate

Oxygen, Antioxidant, or Hydrating Facial: To restore, hydrate, and nourish damaged and dehydrated skin

Paraffin Mask Facial: To penetrate ingredients to promote hydration, softening with an occlusive paraffin mask

Sensitive Skin Facial: To soothe and calm sensitive skin[3]

focus on specific goals or the addition of specialty treatments or products into the basic template that achieve excellence.

Let us discuss a client who has come into your clinic with acne and oily and problematic skin. You may wish to focus on extractions and masking options to address overactive sebaceous glands versus a stimulating massage, which would be counterproductive to your original goal of addressing the underlying problem of oil production. On the other hand, you may have a client who has sought treatments for dry and dehydrated conditions, directing your attention away from the extraction phase of the facial to the treat and correct phase, perhaps using ampoules combined with iontophoresis, targeting the goals at hand.

Professional presentation is important for client satisfaction. Clients will form opinions of what type of service they will be receiving in the first few seconds of meeting you. When working as a professional, you must project a positive image and good hygiene. The pride you take in your appearance is a direct reflection of the pride you take in your work. In addition, the appearance and cleanliness of your work area is especially important. The work area must be clean and organized so you are able to work efficiently and productively. Being prepared also saves time and promotes good customer service. In today's competitive market, presentation is very important, and a negative first impression could be your last opportunity with this client. With today's consumer, worried about diseases and bloodborne pathogens, even a dust ball in the corner can be a red flag. It is important to do a walk-through of your facility, viewing it from a client's perspective.

Suggested Steps for a Machine Facial

1. *Light cleansing*—Removal of all makeup and preparation for skin analysis.
   a. Remove eye makeup and lipstick with cotton rounds saturated with makeup remover or cleanser.
   b. Remove face makeup with a cleansing lotion. Rinse with sponges or warm moist towels.
   c. Wipe face with cotton pads soaked in toner.
2. *Analysis and consultation*—Establish skin type and conditions to determine treatment.
   a. Place moistened eye pads on eyes.
   b. Examine skin under a magnifying lamp held 6 to 12 inches from the skin. Observe for the following:
      (1) Skin's general condition and skin problems, e.g., acne, rosacea, or sensitivity
      (2) Color and texture of the skin and areas of pigmentation
      (3) Pore size, comedones or blocked pores, or papules
      (4) Areas of excess oil or dry flaky patches
      (5) Loss of elasticity
      (6) Dilated capillaries
   c. Turn off lights and examine skin under Wood's lamp.
   d. Discuss the results of the analysis with client. Make notes on facial analysis chart or at the end of the treatment. This would also be an appropriate time to recommend any home-care products that would be effective and to discuss a treatment plan or proceed directly into the facial process.
3. *Deep cleansing, exfoliation, and extractions*—Deeper cleansing, exfoliation of the buildup of dead skin cells, and extraction of comedones.
   a. Turn steamer on. Keep 15 to 18 inches from the face. Steam may be omitted according to skin type, conditions, and sensitivity.
   b. Apply deep cleansing product to face.
   c. Cleanse with a rotating brush. For sensitive skin, use a deep cleansing massage instead.
   d. Remove solution with sponges or warm towels. At this point, you may use the vacuum attachment to remove any superficial debris or use after the disincrustation phase.
   e. At this stage, if there are oily areas or clogged pores, disincrustation (facilitating deep pore cleansing by the use of galvanic current) may be used prior to extractions.
      (1) Apply disincrustation solution to T-zone area. If the skin is dry or dehydrated, do not do disincrustation.
      (2) Have the client hold the ground to galvanic current machine (it should be covered with a moistened cloth).
      (3) Dip the gauze covered electrode in disincrustation solution and place on the skin, move the electrode, and turn on the machine. Move along forehead, nose, chin, and jaw. Some manufacturers suggest to steam during this procedure as well.
      (4) Rinse with sponges or warm towels.
   f. Place moistened eye pads on eyes.
   g. Move magnifying lamp over face.
   h. Perform extraction, using light pressure with a moist cotton or comedone extractor tool.
   i. Rinse skin with warm water.

    j. Apply high frequency for five minutes. (A cotton round saturated with toner may be used in place of the high frequency.)

4. *Treat and correct*—Corrective treatment for specialized skin conditions. Treatment depends on the skin condition and should be performed following the manufacturer's instructions. This would be an appropriate time to apply an ampoule with light effleurage movements and penetrate by ionto-phoresis (the introduction of ions by means of galvanic current). Remember, whenever disincrustation is used, to follow with iontophoresis to rebalance the skin.

5. *Massage*—Offers relaxation to client and stimulates blood and lymph circulation and cell turnover. Use the massage technique appropriate to skin type. If the client has fragile skin, omit the massage or opt to use Viennese massage (a type of high frequency application). Lymphatic drainage massage may also be used during this stage in place of the Viennese massage.

6. *Mask*—Places concentrated nutrients on the skin for an extended period of time to help correct the skin.

    a. Choose a mask that is appropriate for the skin type.

    b. Prepare the mask in a small bowl.

    c. Apply with a clean brush at medium thickness, using upward strokes and avoiding the eyes and nose membranes. Steam may also be used during this step, depending on the manufacturer's instructions, which are included with the mask. Remember not to over steam the skin.

    d. Place eye pads on the eyes and leave on the face for 10 to 15 minutes.

    e. Rinse thoroughly with sponges or warm moist towels.

7. *Completion*—Restoring and rebalancing the skin. Discuss home skin care regimen.

    a. Apply freshener.

    b. Apply eye cream.

    c. Apply light moisturizer. (Some manufacturers also suggest using high frequency to penetrate creams at this juncture in the protocol.)

    d. Apply sunscreen.

    e. Discuss home skin care regimen.

    f. Schedule client's next appointment.

■ OBSERVING THE SKIN

magnifying lamp

an illuminated lamp combined with a magnification lens that magnifies the client's skin, assisting the aesthetician in the analysis portion of the facial treatment

Wood's lamp

a black light that reveals variation in skin color according to skin condition and is used during the skin analysis portion of a facial treatment

It is important to observe the skin thoroughly, using both a **magnifying lamp** and a **Wood's lamp**. Observation under the magnifying lamp determines overall skin texture, tissue elasticity, and visible conditions. The Wood's lamp shows different skin conditions that reveal **hyperpigmentation** and **hypopigmentation**, oiliness, sun damage, or dehydration. This information should be recorded on the treatment form at the end of the treatment with other treatment or home-care notes. Observation should continue throughout the treatment by noting how the skin responds to products, massage, and the overall facial.

    There are three levels of gathering information that are important for a proper skin analysis: determining the Fitzpatrick type, determining skin

Pretreatment Setup

1. Prepare the facial bed in the following order:
   a. bed warmer
   b. fitted sheet on top of bed warmer
   c. flat sheet draped
   d. light blanket placed over sheet
   e. bath sheet on top of flat sheet, leaving space at top for hand towel
   f. headband positioned on top of towel
   g. cotton towel folded diagonally with points facing out (head wrap)
   h. facial gown folded on top of facial bed
2. Be certain that the room contains every supply that may be needed for the aseptic procedure, such as gloves and EPA approved, hospital grade disinfectant. General supplies used during the treatment should be organized for easy use during the procedure.
3. Place products on the shelf of a cart in an organized fashion. Use small dispensing containers or those with pumps to easily dispense the products.

type based on genetic factors, and observing any existing skin conditions. These can be easily observed under a Wood's lamp. This information is helpful in determining future treatments and home-care regiments. In its simplest form, the Fitzpatrick skin typing is a method of skin typing that measures the amount of pigment in the skin and its tolerance to the sun. (See Figure 8–4.)

Additionally, Fitzpatrick skin typing will predict the skin's response to treatments. (See Tables 8–3, 8–4, 8–5, 8–6, 8–7, and 8–8.) To get to these classifications a number of questions are asked of each patient, together with your own examination. Add up the total scores for each of the three sections for your Skin Type Score. This will give you a better evaluation of your skin type.

hyperpigmentation
overproduction and overdeposits of melanin

hypopigmentation
a lack of pigmentation in the skin

Other Forms of Skin Analysis and Classification

It is important for an aesthetician to master the basics of a facial by practicing the step-by-step movements in sequence and to have an

Suggested Steps for a European Facial (Manual Facial)

Note: European-based facials include the face, neck, and décolleté in most of the steps.

1. *Light cleansing*—Removal of all makeup and preparation for skin analysis.
2. *Analysis and consultation*—Establish skin type and conditions to determine treatment.
3. *Deep cleansing and exfoliation*—Deeper cleansing, exfoliation of the buildup of dead skin cells, and extraction of comedones.
   a. Option 1: Apply deep cleansing solution to the face.
   b. Option 2: Perform a second or extended cleansing with a milky cleanser.
   c. Option 3: If you have an exfoliation mask such as an enzyme that may require processing time, a nice relaxing massage can be performed on the foot and legs. If you want to further pamper the client, you may also add heated foot booties after the massage sequence. Reflexology may be substituted at this time.
   d. Remove with sponges or warm towels.
   e. Apply an antiseptic toner.
4. *Massage and corrective treatment*—Delivers specialized ingredients, offers relaxation to the client, stimulates blood and lymph circulation and cell turnover. In European facials the massage phase can be used in two ways. In oily or congested skin types, an alkaline-based massage cream with stimulating massage movements may be used to loosen debris and comedones for easy removal during extractions. For skin types that are dryer, creams that are hydrating and heavier will be used. Steam is usually used with these types of massages.
   a. Apply a massage cream appropriate to the skin type. Use the massage technique appropriate to skin type. Omit the massage if the client's skin is fragile.
   b. Remove cream with sponges or a warm moist towel.
   c. Place moistened eye pads on eyes.
   d. Move magnifying lamp over face.
   e. Perform extraction using light pressure with moist cotton or a comedone extractor tool.
   f. Rinse skin with warm water.
   g. Apply a toner or corrective treatment.
5. *Mask*—Places concentrated nutrients on the skin for an extended period of time to help correct the skin.
6. Choose a mask that is appropriate for the skin type.
   a. Prepare the mask in a small bowl.
   b. Apply with a clean brush at medium thickness, using upward strokes and avoiding the eyes and nose membranes. An eye and lip treatment may be integrated at this time by applying specialized eye and lip serums under a specialized eye and lip mask and covering with cotton pads moistened with toner.
   c. Place eye pads on the eyes and leave on face for 10 to 15 minutes.
   d. At this time a nice relaxing massage can be performed on the hands, arms, and shoulders. If you want to further pamper the client, you may also add heated hand mitts after the massage sequence. Reflexology may be substituted at this time.

e. Rinse thoroughly with sponges or warm moist towels.

7. *Completion*—Restoring and rebalancing the skin. Discussing home skin care regimen.

a. Apply toner.

b. Apply eye cream.

c. Apply light moisturizer.

d. Apply sunscreen.

e. Discuss home skin care regimen.

f. Schedule client's next appointment.

understanding of the protocol, the products, and the tools used. (See Figure 8–5.) Assessing the client's skin type and skin conditions is a crucial part of the process. An aesthetician must be well versed in this in order to proceed with proper treatment and product use.

Products Used in a Facial

Products used in a facial should be directly associated with the skin type and condition to achieve optimal results. It is important to remember that

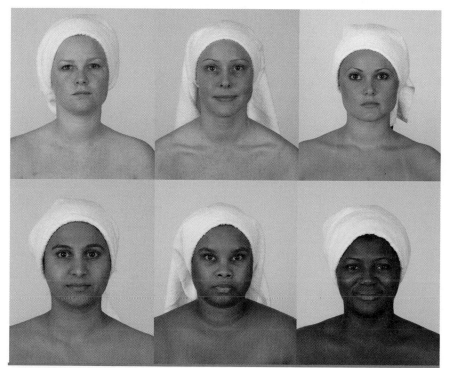

Figure 8–4 Fitzpatrick skin typing allows a clinician to predict the response to treatment

Table 8–3 Fitzpatrick Skin Typing Scale

Skin Type	Skin Color	Hair & Eye Color	Reaction to Sun	Common Ethnic Considerations
Type I	White	Blond hair & green eyes	Always burns, freckles	English, Scottish
Type II	White	Blond hair & green/blue eyes	Always burns, freckles, difficult to tan	Northern European
Type III	White	Blond/brown hair & blue/brown eyes	Tans after several burns, may freckle	German
Type IV	Brown	Brown hair & brown eyes	Tans more than average, rarely burns, rarely freckles	Mediterranean, Southern European, Hispanic
Type V	Dark brown	Brown/black hair & brown eyes	Tans with ease, rarely burns, no freckles	Asian, Indian, some Africans
Type VI	Black	Black hair & brown/black eyes	Tans, never burns, deeply pigmented never freckles	Africans

the objective of treatments and home-care regimes is to bring the skin back to normalcy. Each manufacturer has a variety of products within its lines, but there are some basic commonalities among them.

The makeup removers used today are relatively the same. Differences, however, are more noticeable with cleansers, toners, moisturizers, masks, and other specialty products. For this reason, it is best to think in

Table 8–4 Genetic Disposition[4]

	0	1	2	3	4	Score
What color are your eyes?	Light blue, gray, green	Blue, gray, or green	Blue	Dark brown	Brownish black	
What is the natural color of your hair?	Sandy red	Blond	Chestnut/dark blond	Dark brown	Black	
What color is your skin (nonexposed areas)?	Reddish	Very pale	Pale with beige tint	Light brown	Dark brown	
Do you have freckles on unexposed areas?	Many	Several	Few	Incidental	None	
					Genetic disposition total	

Table 8-5   Reaction to Sun Exposure[5]

	0	1	2	3	4	Score
What happens when you stay too long in the sun?	Painful redness, blistering, peeling	Blistering followed by peeling	Burns sometimes followed by peeling	Rare burns	Never had burns	
To what degree do you turn brown?	Hardly or not at all	Light color tan	Reasonable tan	Tan very easily	Turn dark brown quickly	
Do you turn brown with several hours of sun exposure?	Never	Seldom	Sometimes	Often	Always	
How does your face react to the sun?	Very sensitive	Sensitive	Normal	Very resistant	Never had a problem	
					Reaction to sun exposure total	

Table 8-6   Tanning Habits[6]

	1	2	3	4	5	Score
When did you last expose your body to sun (or artificial sunlamp/tanning cream)?	More than 3 months ago	2–3 months ago	1–2 months ago	Less than a month ago	Less than 2 weeks ago	
Did you expose the area to be treated to the sun?	Never	Hardly ever	Sometimes	Often	Always	
					Tanning habits total	

Table 8-7   Scores[7]

Summary
Total for genetic disposition
Total for reaction to sun exposure
Total for tanning habits
Skin Type Score

Table 8–8	Your Fitzpatrick Skin Type[8]
Skin Type Score	**Fitzpatrick Skin Type**
0–7	I
8–16	II
17–25	III
25–30	IV
Over 30	V–VI

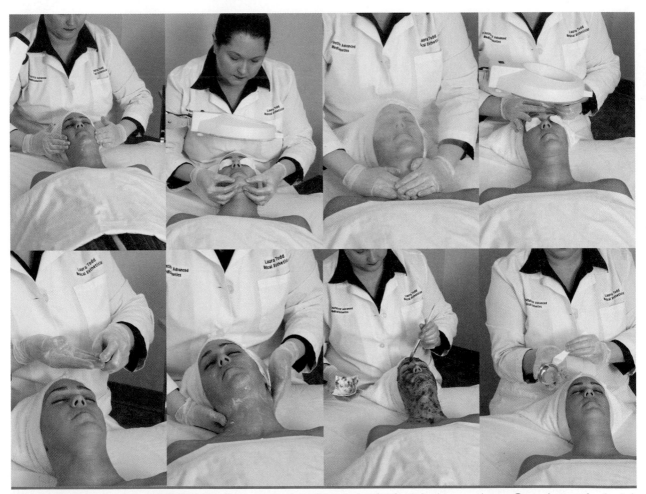

Figure 8–5 Step one of a facial: the first cleansing. Step two of a facial: skin analysis. Step three of a facial: deep cleansing and exfoliation with steam. Step three of a facial: extractions. Step four of a facial: application of a specialty serum during the treat and correct phase. Step five of a facial: relaxing massage. Step six of a facial: the application of a mask in the facial process. Step seven of a facial: completion with the application of a moisturizer with an SPF.

Glogau Classifications of Photodamage

The Glogau Photodamage Classification system presents four levels of photo damage.

Type I: No wrinkles at rest or while moving

Early photoaging

Mild pigment changes

No keratosis

Minimal to no wrinkles

20s to 30s or younger

Minimal acne scarring can be seen if present

No to minimal makeup necessary

Type II: Wrinkles only in motion, visible when the person is talking, laughing, frowning, etc.

Early-to-moderate photoaging

Lentigines, other pigment changes showing

Wrinkles forming

Light keratosis

Nasolabial lines beginning to form

30s to 40s

Minimal makeup

Type III: Wrinkles at rest—you see the wrinkles when the person is not moving

Advanced photoaging

Hyperpigmentation

Telangiectasia

Keratosis

Wrinkles even when not moving

40s to 50s

Makeup always worn

Acne scarring, when present, shows through makeup

Type IV: Wrinkles as predominant characteristic; you see only wrinkles

Severe photoaging

Sallow-ashy skin color

Prior skin cancers

Wrinkles all over

Makeup not worn, sets in cracks

Severe acne scarring

Rubin's Classification of Photodamage

Dermatologist Mark G. Rubin has created a method for determining the level of photodamage.[9] The categories are as follows:

Level 1

Alterations are in the epidermis only. These changes are primarily superficial pigment changes, roughness, lentigines, a dull or ashy appearance, and increased thickness.

This client will benefit from a superficial peeling such as glycolic acid and a steady home-care program combining AHA and/or BHAs, nourishers, antioxidants, and sunscreens.

Level 2

Alterations are in the epidermis and papillary dermis. These conditions may include all of those seen in level I, as well as actinic keratosis, stronger pigmentation values, flat seborrheic keratosis, and an increase in wrinkles.

This client will benefit from medium-depth peels such as TCA (trichloracetic acid) and a more aggressive home-care program including retinoids and hydroquinone.

(Continued)

Level 3

Changes are not only in the epidermis and papillary dermis but also in the reticular dermis. This will be the severest level of photodamage, and skin will be leathery, will be yellow in color, and will exhibit open comedones.

This client likely would benefit from laser resurfacing and possibly other cosmetic procedures along with a progressive home-care program depending upon age and sensitivity to performance and active agents.

Kligman Rosacea Classification

Dermatologists Albert M. Kligman and Gerd Plewig developed a method for classifying rosacea.

Stage I

Erythema in the areas of the nasolabial folds, cheeks, and glabellum (forehead). Skin seems to itch and burn in the presence of cosmetics.

Stage II

Inflammation, pustules, and papules are present, and pores seem larger; condition may spread over other parts of the face including hairline and chin.

Stage III

The most serious form of rosacea, large nodules present, orange-peel and coarse appearance.

Kligman Acne Classification

Dermatologists Albert M. Kligman and Gerd Plewig developed a method for classifying acne.

Grade I

Open and closed comedones with transitory blemishes.

Grade II

Larger open and closed comedones, a small number of pustules and papules.

Grade III

Many open and closed comedones, pustules, and papules, several cystic lesions, pigment changes, and inflamed erythema (redness) where the area is painful.

Grade IV

Includes all of the above combined with advanced stages of cystic acne, scarring, inflammation, and erythema (redness).

terms of dryness or oiliness or degrees of sensitivity, and to lean toward prominent indicators when choosing a product.

Cleansers   Most product lines address the following three skin types with their cleansers:

- normal to dry
- combination to oily
- sensitive

Normal to dry skin types prefer a creamy cleanser. Oily skin types benefit from a gel base or foaming cleanser that contains ingredients to address the excess sebum. Combination skin types can benefit from either, depending on the degree to which they are dry or oily. A foaming cleanser may be too drying or a cream-based one not effective enough. While it is a personal preference to a point, certain considerations must be evaluated. Among them are skin type and skin condition, as well as any allergies or skin sensitivities that the client might have.

As with all skin types, there is a point where any product with a pH that is too acidic or alkaline can be too harsh and strip the natural balance of the **acid mantle**. The acid mantle is composed of sebum and sweat, and is considered to be the protective barrier of our skin, protecting us from certain types of bacteria and microorganisms. In the case of oily skin and harsh cleansers, a rebound effect can occur. This is seen in **acneic** conditions, when the skin has been dried out to extremes. In these instances, the skin works overtime to produce sebum in an effort to rebalance the skin. This contributes to an increase in the number of breakouts and can cause sensitivity that further inflames the condition. Products that contain heavy creams or ingredients that are comedogenic can aggravate oily and acneic skin conditions.

Toners, Astringents, and Fresheners   Toners, astringents, and fresheners also have a hierarchy that ranges from sensitive to dry to oily. Typically an astringent is the strongest, a toner is somewhat milder, and a freshener is the gentlest. Astringents are stronger than fresheners and toners and are usually reserved for oily or acneic clients. Toners are frequently used for all types, though there may be a slight adjustment in the ingredients from dry to oily. Fresheners are frequently used for sensitive skin conditions.

Intensive Products, Ampoules, or Serums   Intensive treatments can encompass ampoules or serums to address specific targets, such as collagen ampoules for hydration, firming ampoules for elasticity issues, skin lighting and brightening ampoules for hyperpigmentation, antioxidant cocktails for premature aging and sun damaged types, oil controlling ampoules for acneic conditions, or calming ampoules for rosacea. Ampoules or serums are usually more expensive in the product line because they contain a greater percent and concentration of results-oriented ingredients. These products can be added into the treat and correct phase of the facial treatment.

Massage Oils and Creams   A massage is most often performed during the relaxation phase of a facial treatment unless the skin is extremely

---

acid mantle
The acid mantle is composed of sebum and sweat, and is considered to be the protective barrier of our skin protecting us from certain types of bacteria and microorganisms

acneic
having acne condition

toners, astringents, and fresheners
have a hierarchy that ranges from sensitive to dry to oily. Typically an astringent is the strongest, a toner is somewhat milder, and a freshener is the gentlest. Astringents are stronger than fresheners and toners and are usually reserved for oily or acneic clients.

sensitive, is severely acneic, or has other contraindicative conditions. The decision to use a massage oil or cream is a personal preference.

Most product lines specifically manufacture facial massage oils and creams, so they are therefore noncomedogenic. The oils may not be a good choice for clients with oily skin types who may need a lighter massage cream. Dry and dehydrated skin types benefit from either due to the hydration that both can provide. Many aestheticians may opt to combine the application of ampoules and serums in with the massage, depending on the chosen facial protocol.

Masks   Masks come in the following three forms:

- gel
- cream
- clay

Gel-based masks are very hydrating and are commonly used after microdermabrasion or a light chemical exfoliation. They can be used on all skin types. Cream-based masks are nondrying and usually have calming and hydrating properties. Clay masks are used on oily and acneic skin conditions to dry the excess sebum. Some may contain added ingredients, such as sulfur, to address acne.

Moisturizers   Skin type determines the level of moisture that needs to be considered. Clients with oily skin still need hydration and prefer a lighter moisturizer specifically designed for their skin type. They may also benefit from a moisturizer that hydrates and controls oil.

Dry and dehydrated skin types will benefit from a very emollient moisturizer that restores the skin to normalcy. Moisturizers designed for sensitive skin may be fragrance-free and dermatologist tested. Sensitive skin moisturizers may also have calming and soothing botanicals. Some product lines also have moisturizers to address conditions such as acne or rosacea.

The most important thing to remember is that the analysis of the client and the choice of products used relates directly to the end result. (See Table 8–9.) Aestheticians who do not have a solid foundation of skin analysis and consultation skills will not deliver optimal results.

■ HYDRATING FACIALS

hydrating facials
restore moisture to the skin and are beneficial for dehydrated skin types

Hydrating facials can assist with the symptoms of dry skin and help elevate dehydrated skin by adding moisture and bringing the skin into balance. These facials usually contain calming and soothing agents as

Table 8–9   Products and Their Functions

Product	Function
Eye makeup remover	• Dissolves pigmented products around eyes and lips, yet is gentle for delicate eye area • Softens and moisturizes delicate eye area • Nongreasy formulas are good for contact lens wearers
Cleanser	• Dissolves makeup • Dissolves oil and surface impurities • Has nondetergent cleansing ability
Washable or foaming cleanser	• Acts like soap with a foaming cleansing feel • Cleanses skin without the harshness of soap • Is nonalkalinic and easy to use
Freshener or toner	• Removes traces of makeup and cleanser • Readjusts the skin's pH level • Refreshes skin to feel completely clean • Provides moisture • Prepares the skin for application of correction fluid or day or night cream
Day cream	• Protects and nourishes the skin • Softens and moisturizes skin • Provides smooth base for subsequent application of makeup
Sunscreen	• Protects the skin from harmful ultraviolet rays • Some contain moisturizers
Night cream	• Nourishes the skin • Feeds special treatment ingredients into the skin during sleep • Softens and moisturizes skin
Mask	• Blankets the skin to provide special moisture and other performance ingredients • Draws and lifts impurities and/or dead cells • Tightens and tones

well. The important follow-up to this treatment is proper home care and maintaining the results that have been achieved.

The components of a facial that make it hydrating are related to the addition of specific products, such as a hydrating ampoule, a moisturizer, or a hydrating mask. One of the most popular hydrating masks is a gel mask. The gel mask can be used on all skin types and conditions as it is very gentle and hydrating. The use of galvanic current or iontophoresis during a facial can also be a nice addition to ensure penetration of a specialty serum or ampoule. Paraffin masks, which are also used to help penetrate and moisturize the skin, are not suitable for oily skin as they may be too stimulating. Exfoliation (AHA, enzymes) may also be effective for these conditions as the removal of built-up skin cells provides better product penetration.

Candidates for a Hydrating Facial

Dry skin may occur due to daily activities such as bathing or showering with hot temperatures and vigorous scrubbing with washcloths or harsh soaps that temporarily remove the skin's oily lipid layer causing moisture loss, which can lead to dehydrated skin. Dry skin can also occur as a result of genetics, thyroid disease, or excessive weight loss, or as a part of the normal aging process yielding a decrease in sebum production. Symptoms include a feeling of tightness or tautness (especially after showering), a loss of plumpness and luster, redness, or a rougher texture. Dry areas may result in the skin becoming red and itchy, leading to dermatitis or cracks and fissures. In advanced cases of dry skin, or as with xerosis, dry skin becomes a long-term problem recurring often, especially in the winter. Ichthyosis is a skin disorder inherited from one or both parents, which causes the formation of dry, fish-like scales on the skin's surface. The condition often begins in early childhood and is usually lifelong. Dry skin benefits from water-in-oil moisturizer, which will tend to be heavier and richer than others. A must-have component in a dry skin client's home-care regimen is a product that is effective in sealing in the moisture once it has been introduced.

Dehydrated skin is the result of decreased moisture content in the skin. Signs of dehydrated skin include a dull complexion, redness, and skin tightness, patches of sensitivity, blotchiness, and flaky skin. An important concept to remember as an aesthetician is that dehydrated skin lacks moisture, whereas dry skin lacks oil or sebum. Unlike dry skin, it is not due to heredity, aging, or temporary loss of the lipid layer. As such, treatment for the two conditions should differ. Temporary dehydration can occur as a result of the loss of the skin's lipid layer, as previously discussed with dry skin conditions, and can resolve itself when the culprits are removed from the client's daily regime. Dehydra-

---

> A hydrating facial restores moisture to the skin and is beneficial for dehydrated skin types.

dry skin
a condition resulting from a decrease in sebum production

dehydrated skin
the result of decreased moisture content in the skin

tion may be attributed to seasonal changes, other environmental factors such as sun or wind exposure, lack of water intake, climate changes such as those found in the dry air desert states, air travel, and heating units or dehumidifiers—all of which can steal the skin's moisture. Even people with oily skin types can suffer from dehydrated skin. With oily-dehydrated skin types, take care to use a light hydrating moisturizer.

Suggested Steps for a Hydrating Facial for Dry Skin

1. *Light cleansing*
2. *Analysis and consultation*
3. *Deep cleansing, exfoliation*—For extremely dry skin, steam may be omitted.
4. *Treat and correct*—Corrective treatment for specialized skin conditions. This would be an appropriate time to apply an ampoule with light effleurage movements and or penetrate by iontophoresis (the introduction of ions by means of a galvanic current).
5. *Massage*—For extremely dry or fragile skin you may omit the massage or opt for a Viennese massage (a type of high frequency application where the client holds the high frequency electrode with both hands while the technician performs a massage).
6. *Hydrating Mask Options*
   a. *Gel Mask*
      (1) Apply a hydrating gel mask with a brush, using upward strokes and avoiding the eyes and the nose membranes. Place eye pads on the eyes and leave on the face for 10 to 15 minutes.
      (2) Rinse thoroughly with sponges or warm moist towels.
      (3) Wipe face with cotton pads soaked in hydrating toner.
   b. *Hydrating Paraffin Mask* (may be used instead of a gel mask)
      (1) Apply an eye and lip gel. Apply eye pads over the eye area.
      (2) Dip cotton gauze or paraffin strips into the paraffin bath.
      (3) Wipe excess with a wooden spatula. Apply three or four layers.
      (4) Process for 15 minutes. For a greater hydrating effect, apply an ampoule or serum under the mask.
      (5) Remove the mask and rinse thoroughly with sponges or warm moist towels.
      (6) Wipe face with cotton pads soaked in a hydrating toner.
7. *Completion*

Avoid rich or heavy moisturizing creams. Dehydrated skin can benefit from oil-in-water moisturizers, which tend to be lighter than the water-in-oil moisturizers previously recommended for dry skin types. Dehydrated skin can be easily restored and prevented. Dry skin is an ongoing condition where symptoms need to be evaluated and reevaluated.[10]

> Dehydrated skin lacks moisture, whereas dry skin lacks oil or sebum. As such, treatment for the two conditions should differ.

What Can Be Expected from a Hydrating Facial

A hydrating facial will give the client temporary relief from dehydrated skin including a dull complexion, redness, skin tightness, patches of sensitivity, blotchiness, and flaky skin. The main focus for the aesthetician is to determine what factors have caused this condition and how to prevent an environment that allows for dehydration. In certain instances, such as a client's living in arid climates or working as a flight attendant, the client is continually exposed to drier air conditions, and the only resolutions would be increasing the water uptake and addressing the symptoms of the dehydrated skin with hydrating facials and serums or creams that can be taken home to extend the benefits of the facial treatment.

A hydrating facial comes in many forms. Some hydrating facials include specialty hydrating masks, the integration of hydrating products throughout the entire facial process, and the use of machines such as ultrasound or iontophoresis (galvanic current) to penetrate ampoules, creams, or hydrating ingredients. The protocol provides an example of how you may integrate products and technologies to achieve a hydrating facial.

■ ADVANCED FACIAL TREATMENTS

Ultrasound

In a physical therapy setting, ultrasound is used to stimulate blood flow, increase metabolic rate, and warm up tissues to promote temporary pain relief. Ultrasound used for cosmetic application has increasingly gained popularity. Its current applications include its use to penetrate products or provide deep cleansing action. (See Figure 8–6.) For the purpose of deep cleansing action, a spatula-like handpiece is used in conjunction with water-based cleansers and steam to perform a deep cleansing. It is believed that the ultrasound assists in dislodging any surface contaminants or impurities embedded in the follicles. In the case of product penetration, a circular flat handpiece or the opposite side of the spatula is used in conjunction with serums and ampoules for deeper penetration of products.

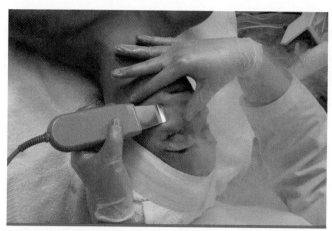

Figure 8–6 The use of an ultrasonic machine will improve the results of a facial

When ascertaining the proper application parameters for the cosmetic application of ultrasound, it is first important to understand that the depth of tissue penetration is not intensity dependent, but frequency dependent. Cosmetic application usually consists of a tissue penetration depth of less than two centimeters that can be obtained by using a three-megahertz frequency. Most of the ultrasonic energy with a three-megahertz frequency will be absorbed in the superficial tissue. In contrast, the slower, one-megahertz frequency will have less energy absorbed superficially, allowing for deeper penetration, and will heat tissue up to three to five centimeters deep.

One important aspect to remember is that if the ultrasound is placed directly on one part of the skin for too long, the excessive heat buildup can cause unstable cavitation. During treatments it is important to remember that the technician should maintain constant movement of the handpiece on moist tissue. There are contraindications to damaged or thin fragile skin, and ultrasound should never perform close to the eye area. Other contraindications include clients with heart conditions, pacemakers, or electrical implants, pregnant women, or clients with diabetes.

Light Therapy

Pioneered by Patrick Bitter Jr., MD, Intense Pulsed Light (IPL) or photorejuvenation treatments use a noncoherent, broadband, pulsed light source to treat vascular and pigmented lesions of the skin. His studies evaluated the role of intense pulsed light in the rejuvenation of photoaged skin. IPL skin treatments use specific wavelengths of light to achieve what is called "photorejuvenation" and is sometimes referred to as a photofacial or fotofacial. (See Figure 8–7.) The term "photorejuvenation" refers to the nonablative or nonvaporizing treatment of skin cells to address skin

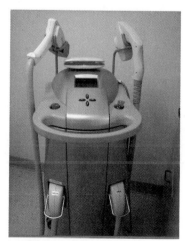

Figure 8–7 An IPL machine is a useful tool in conjunction with a facial

Suggested Steps for an Ultrasound Facial Treatment for Deep Cleansing and Product Penetration

Supplies:

Typical table, client draping and linen setup

Gloves

Gauze pads or cotton rounds

Sponges (disposable)

Water bowl

Eye pads for client

Water-based cleanser

Treatment mask (optional)

Massage cream

Toner

Specialty serums or ampoules

Moisturizing sunscreen (SPF 15 minimum)

Procedure:

Deep pore cleansing and mild exfoliation for the facial area:

1. Drape client and secure hair away from the face.
2. Perform a precleansing and remove makeup.
3. Apply cleanser combined with a small trace of water for moisture and apply to the face in small circular motions, leaving that area lightly wet. (A mild disincrustation fluid may also be used in severely oily and congested skin types.)
4. Steam may be used to maintain moisture at this time. If you do not want to use steam, use a gauze pad or sponge to rewet any drying areas as needed. Do not use ultrasonic handpieces on dry skin. Discontinue treatment if the client feels any discomfort at any time.
   a. In performing the treatments it is preferred to move from forehead to right side of the face to left side of the face, and then proceed to upper lip and chin area. Isolate the area in which you wish to begin your treatment and gently secure/stretch the skin to be treated between your thumb and pointer finger as typically used when performing a microdermabrasion treatment. Holding the handpiece facing downward at a 45° angle, gently glide it across the skin surface in a light back and forth pressing movement (similar to scraping paint but without the pressure). Increase or decrease intensity as indicated by the manufacturer.
   b. Rinse with sponges and/or warm towel.
5. Deep hydration and penetration of serums for the facial area:
   a. Apply desired product to be penetrated.
   b. In performing the treatments it is preferred to move from forehead to right side of the face to left side of the face then proceed to upper lip and chin area. Isolate the area in which you wish to begin your treatment and gently secure/stretch the skin to be treated between your thumb and pointer finger as typically used when performing a microdermabrasion treatment. Holding the handpiece facing downward at a 45° angle, gently glide it across the skin surface in a light back and forth pressing movement (similar to scraping paint but without the pressure). If available, a penetration handpiece will be used in circular motions and as directed by the manufacturer. Increase or decrease intensity as indicated by the manufacturer. Apply serum as needed to maintain moisture level.
6. Finish with a moisturizer of your choice and SPF.

irregularities. Photorejuvenation is typically used to treat a wide variety of benign conditions such as vascular lesions, pigmented lesions, and skin laxity. Aging, sun exposure, and other factors can cause the appearance of broken capillaries and blood vessels on the face also known as telangiectasia, or spider veins. Rosacea is also a common skin condition noted to respond well to IPL. In the case of lax skin and loss of tonicity, the IPL treats imperfections in the superficial layers of the skin, while delivering thermal energy to deeper tissues. It is believed this energy has an effect on collagen production and helps to firm and tighten the skin.

On average, four to six treatments are recommended, scheduled at three-week intervals. Each session usually lasts about 20 minutes. Assessments of clients will include the use of the Fitzpatrick skin scale to determine if they are candidates for the treatment. Other advanced skin typing mechanisms may also be used including Glogau or Rubin's classification of photodamage, and, in the case of rosacea or acne, the Kligman classifications may be used. When determining treatment parameters, remember that the longer wavelengths are used to rejuvenate and smooth the skin, and the shorter wavelengths are used for pigmented and vascular lesions. Before treatment, a cold gel is applied to the areas to be treated and clients put on protective eyewear. During treatment, the technician gently applies the smooth, glass filter (specific to the desired target) surface of the IPL handpiece to the skin. Light is delivered to the skin surface in precise pulses to the area being treated. Results from a full series of treatments usually last for a year or more. The technician also wears protective eyewear and in some cases a smoke evacuator is also recommended to eliminate any plume that may be produced by hair that may be present. IPL may also be used for hair reduction/removal.

LED (light emitting diode) photorejuvenation is rated as a Class I or II device by the FDA, depending on the model, and uses one or more individual wavelengths of light delivered at a low intensity. One popular treatment range is red light (625 to 765 nm) combined with invisible infrared light (880 to 920 nm). It is noted for its effects on stimulating metabolism and cellular turnover for mature skin. The benefits from this type of light therapy are thought to stem from an increase in cellular efficiency and may stimulate ATP (adenosine triphosphate) release, which allows cells to accept nutrients and get rid of waste faster. This treatment is typically performed as a series of 12 treatments and is not as powerful as the IPL. It is usually delivered by rotating a small handpiece over the face for specified intervals. It is important to always avoid the thyroid area during treatments and to ensure the client is wearing protective eyewear. New technology has emerged that allows this light therapy to be delivered in the form of a rotating panel and is geared toward ease of use for the aesthetician.

Other forms of light therapy may also be found in water therapy capsule devises that emit different ranges of the spectrum in a treatment to encourage a sense of well-being. Light therapy will definitely be a centerpiece for estheticians for years to come.[11]

Non-Laser- and Non-Light-Based Methods of Removing Skin Imperfections

Based on the electrical current used by an electrologist stemmed a method to remove small spider veins on the body, facial telangiectasia, cherry angiomas, skin tags, and vascular blemishes. Technologies currently

---

Suggested Steps for a LED or Photorejuvenation Facial Treatment

Supplies:

Typical table, client draping and linen setup	Water-based cleanser
	Massage cream
Gloves	Toner
Gauze pads or cotton rounds	Specialty serums or ampoules
Sponges (disposable)	Moisturizing sunscreen
Water bowl	(SPF 15 minimum)
Eye pads for client	LED machine

Procedure:

1. Drape client and secure hair away from the face.
2. Perform a precleansing and remove makeup.
3. Perform a second cleansing and apply toner with cotton rounds.
4. Apply a serum or ampoule of your choice.
5. Use protective eyewear on the client and cover the thyroid area.
6. Position the unit if you have an automatic pane or, if you have a manual handpiece, rotate the small handpiece over the face for specified intervals.
   a. In performing the treatments it is preferred to move from forehead to right side of the face to left side of the face then proceed to upper lip and chin area.
   b. Apply serum as needed to maintain moisture level.
7. Finish the treatment with an ampoule or cream of your choice, and end with a draining massage.
8. Apply SPF.

used integrate low levels of radio frequency (RF) and direct current (DC) to electrocoagulate capillaries. The treatment is vessel specific and results in minimal skin reaction or collateral tissue damage. The units use an external probe and conducting gel to conduct the energy on the surface of the skin. As a result, there is no actual skin penetration, just a light touch of the probe on the epidermis. The probes vary in size, smaller for the facial area and larger for the body areas. The typical probe uses an ultrafine insulated nonpenetrating probe, allowing application of the treatment while still protecting surrounding tissue.

The procedure starts with a thorough cleansing of the area with an antiseptic. Anesthesia can be applied to the area to be treated and, if desired, should be done so at least 30 minutes before the procedure. In the DC mode, the client must hold a ground as with galvanic facial therapies. A conductive gel is applied with a cotton swab and the sterile probe is placed on the surface of the skin at the target area. Low-level RF and DC pass through the probe to the vessel or target. The technician will look for blanching of the area during the treatments as a stop point. The blood in the vessel will then be clotted or coagulated, will stop flowing, and will eventually absorb into the surrounding tissue. Posttreatment includes application of an antiseptic, and iontophoresis can be used to calm the area. The treated vessels should not be disturbed for 24 hours. Undue stress can cause renewed blood flow, which may keep the vessel from drying up. The treated vessel should look darker the next day. This is normal and is a good sign that the vessel was properly treated. Skin should not be stretched, and the client should avoid washing the area and exercising for 24 hours. The treated area will form tiny crusts that should fall off in 7 to 10 days. Larger vessels may require more than one treatment. For leg veins, only smaller red or purple veins may be treated; the client may require two or three treatments, and the client should wear support hose or an ace bandage wrap for two days posttreatment. In the case of skin tags the target is the base of the tag just above the skin surface. Tweezers can be used to extend the tag. The mode used for this treatment will consist of radio frequency only. The treatment causes a disruption of blood flow, resulting in the tag dropping off in several days to one week.

Microcurrent

Today many aestheticians are using microcurrent technology in their treatments to reeducate muscles that have lost tonicity due to the effects of aging and gravity. Microcurrent operates on a very low level of current called the microampere (the symbol for microamp is "m"). The microampere is a current of 0.001 ampere or less. This is generally defined as the cosmetic current level. Microcurrent treatments typically use a combination of galvanic and faradic current. These combinations are used for several applications including the deep penetrate serums to hydrate dry and dehydrated skin, stimulate circulation and increase blood flow, and encourage nourishment to deprived tissues as well as microcontractions of the muscles to promote tone and to reeducate lax muscles. It can be an early alternative to Botox in certain instances. The galvanic current is a direct current (DC) and is used in the iontophoresis mode for the penetration of an ionized solution (containing + or − ions) into the surface tissue. The faradic current is a DC galvanic current that is interrupted or alternating, used to affect the tonicity of the muscles by exciting nerves of the peripheral nervous system and produce microcontraction allowing for tightening or relaxation of the muscle. The unit usually has Hz setting, which allows for changes in frequency that are directly connected to the number of microcontractions per second, determining whether the muscle will be relaxed (lengthened) or tightened (shortened). Contraindications include: open wounds, cancerous lesions, heart condition, pacemaker or pacemaker leads, muscular condition, epilepsy, advanced diabetes, hemophilia, pregnancy, as well as newly placed injectable fillers or Botox and implants (seek physician's approval).

The microcurrent units typically come with two handpieces or probes that have receptacles on the ends that allow for the insertion of cotton swabs that are immersed in conductive gel, are applied to the treatment area, and are moved with distinct and very precise directional movements. (See Figure 8–8.) For relaxing protocol movements the probes are usually positioned anatomically at the belly of the muscle and moved toward origin and insertion, resulting in a lengthening of the muscle. For lifting, strengthening, or tightening protocol movements, the probes are positioned at the origin and insertion and moved toward the belly of the muscle, resulting in shortening or compressions of the muscle. There are various other movements that can be administered, depending on the area and issue to be addressed, but typically relaxing and tightening are most prevalent in a treatment sequence.

One of the most popular treatments administered is eyelifting treatments that result in an outcome equivalent to an instant brow lift. If you consider the effects of gravity on the eye area, you can easily visualize which movements would be effective. Consider one of the muscles involved in the eye area, the obicularis oculi muscle; this is the muscle that looks like a circle that surrounds the eye, and it closes the eyelid and compresses the lacrimal sac (tear duct). The treatment that would be most appropriate would be lifting, strengthening, and tightening. Another landmark near this area would be the temporalis muscle. This muscle is

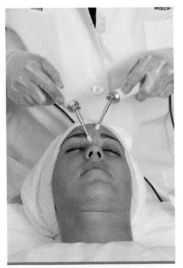

Figure 8–8 Microcurrent technology is used to reeducate muscles that have lost tonicity due to the effects of aging and gravity

responsible for elevating and closing the jaw; it retracts the mandible, clenches the teeth, and draws back the skin of temples. The treatment that would be most appropriate would be lifting, strengthening, and tightening. The goal of microcurrent on these two muscles should be to restore what gravity and time have allowed to droop and become lax. The forehead area is also an area of concern for most. The frontalis muscles lift the eyebrows and result in horizontal (transverse) lines of the forehead. Vertical lines in the forehead region between the eyes (glabellar region) are from the corrugator muscles. The corrugator muscles benefit from relaxing movements in microcurrent treatments. Horizontal wrinkles in this region are from the procerus muscles and also benefit from relaxing treatments. The corrugator and procerus muscles depress and move the eyebrows together. The zygomaticus major is responsible for raising the mouth upward and backward as seen with smiling. The zygomaticus minor is responsible for raising the mouth upward. The risorius is responsible for retracting the mouth. These muscles will show great improvement with a treatment of tightening and strengthening and will decrease the look of marionette lines that are prevalent with aging.

To address the horizontal lines in the forehead area and vertical wrinkles in the glabellar region, relaxing movements during a microcurrent treatment will restore a well-rested, relaxed, and youthful look. Microcurrent treatments are administered in increments of two or three times per week (depending on the severity of the problem) with monthly maintenance treatments once the desired goal is obtained.

■ ANTIOXIDANTS

Free radicals come in the form of a single atom or a group of atoms that has at least one unpaired electron. This unpaired electron results in a highly unstable and highly reactive molecule that tries to gain electrons from neighboring molecules perpetuating a chain or cascading effect.

free radicals
atoms or groups of atoms that have an unpaired electron resulting in a highly unstable molecule

> Muscles that would benefit from lengthening are the anguli oris, buccinator, corrugator, depressor, frontalis, labii inferioris, mentalis, orbicularis oris, and orbicularis oculi.
>
> Muscles that would benefit from tightening or compression are the levator labii superioris nasii, levator labii superioris, platysma, risorius, temporalis, zygomaticus minor, and zygomaticus major.

Suggested Steps for Eye Procedure of the Obicularis Oculi with Microcurrent

Supplies and Setup:

1. General table and draping setup
2. Water and sponges, cotton swabs with paper shaft
3. Gentle cleanser
4. Ionized ampoules solutions
5. Conductive gel
6. Moisturizer and SPF

Procedure:

1. Cleanse the skin and apply the conductive gel along the area you are currently treating. Moisten the cotton swabs that are inserted into the conducting probes. (The gel can serve as a map to remember the area you are working on.)

2. Obicularis oculi area

   a. Set the machine currents to the appropriate levels advised by the manufacturer for the eye area.

   b. Start at the end of the brow closest to the nose, systematically moving toward the end closest to the hairline.

   c. Place one electrode on the very top of the brow at the starting point. Place the other electrode directly below and move electrode toward stationary electrode to pinch together with compression-like movement (your goal is to achieve a half-inch fold of tissue between the tips). Hold for four seconds.

   d. Move horizontally, one cotton swab's space toward the hairline and compress again and hold for four seconds.

   e. Continue to move until you have completed the compression movements along the entire length of the brow.

3. Finish treatment with an eye cream only or a full moisturizing eye treatment.

Free radicals often attack the lipid layer of the skin at the cellular level, impairing the communication functions of the cells. Cellular communication is key to all metabolic processes in the body and free radicals can damage important components of the cell such as DNA. Once the DNA is impaired, so is the genetic code or the blueprint for further cells propagated through mitosis. This degradation in healthy cells is seen in the aging process. The concern aestheticians have is premature aging due to cumulative free radical damage from environmental factors such as cigarette smoke, pollution, radiation, and various chemicals.

Antioxidants neutralize free radicals by donating one of their own electrons, ending the chain reaction. They are stable and do not become free radicals.

Antioxidant nutrients also do not become free radicals when donating an electron because they are stable in either form. Instead they act as scavengers, helping to prevent cell and tissue damage that could lead to cellular damage and disease. Antioxidants can be gained through diets that include foods with manganese, zinc, selenium, vitamin E, vitamin C, and beta-carotene, as well as those with antioxidant enzymes that assist in controlling damage by free radicals.[12]

Candidates for Antioxidant Facials

Candidates for **antioxidant facials** include clients who have prematurely damaged skin due to sun exposure, environmental factors such as cigarette smoke, pollution, radiation, and various chemicals. Almost anyone over 30 could benefit from this type of treatment.

What Can Be Expected from the Use of Antioxidants in a Facial

On a scientific level, immediate benefits from an antioxidant facial cannot really be noticed at the cellular level, and compliance with continued treatments and home care would be the immediate goal of the aesthetician. The immediate benefits at a cosmetic level would be temporary hydration. In general, antioxidant facials we commonly think of focus on the symptoms of the prematurely aged skin. In addition to the treatment, aestheticians should address long term results by focusing on the home-care regiments of clients to ensure that they are using antioxidant creams. They should also inform them of the benefits of dietary and lifestyle changes. Antioxidant products include vitamin C, vitamin E, hyaluronic acid, or other nourishing ingredients.

antioxidant facials
focus on the symptoms of the prematurely aged skin using antioxidant products including vitamin C, vitamin E, hyaluronic acid, or other nourishing ingredients

■ ADDING STEPS TO THE FACIAL

When adding steps into a facial, it is important to determine what the goals are and what needs to be done to achieve them. The change in benefits is directly associated with the products or the machines that are incorporated into the treatment.

Most aestheticians change their results by replacing standard products with ones that are more results oriented and performance based as

Suggested Steps for Antioxidant Facial

1. *Light cleansing*—Removal of all makeup and preparation for skin analysis.
   a. Remove eye makeup and lipstick with cotton rounds.
   b. Remove face makeup with an antioxidant cleansing lotion and rinse with sponges or warm moist towels.
   c. Wipe face with cotton pads soaked in a hydrating antioxidant toner.
2. *Analysis and consultation*
3. *Deep cleansing, exfoliation*
   a. Turn steamer on, keeping 15 to 18 inches from the face.
   b. Apply antioxidant cleanser to the face.
   c. Cleanse with a cleansing massage.
   d. Tissue off or remove solution with sponges or warm towels.
   e. Apply an enzyme mask and process according to the manufacturer's instructions.
   f. Remove solution with sponges or warm towels.
   g. Wipe face with cotton pads soaked in a hydrating antioxidant toner.
4. *Treat and correct*—This would be an appropriate time to apply an antioxidant serum with light effleurage movements and penetrate by iontophoresis (the introduction of ions by means of galvanic current).
5. *Massage*—Massage with an antioxidant massage cream.
6. *Antioxidant Mask*
   a. Apply an antioxidant mask with a brush, using upward strokes and avoiding the eyes and the nose membranes. Place eye pads on the eyes and leave on the face for 10 to 15 minutes.
   b. Rinse thoroughly with sponges or warm moist towels.
   c. Wipe face with cotton pads soaked in a hydrating antioxidant toner.
7. *Completion*

in the case of ampoules or specialty masks. (See Figure 8–9.) One example for a client who has a buildup of excess dead skin cells is replacing exfoliating granules with an enzyme peel. Lymphatic drainage is another step that may be added into the normal facial protocol. Lymphatic drainage is an advanced modality commonly used for detoxification purposes to assist in reducing swelling and to promote healing postsurgery. Because this modality is very advanced in nature, requiring extensive training in

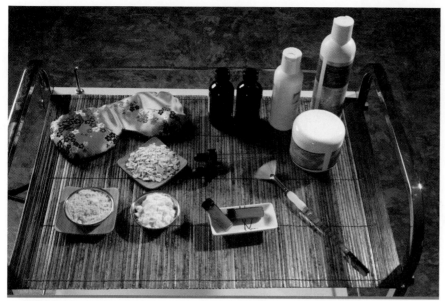

Figure 8–9 Most aestheticians change their results by replacing standard products with ones that are more results oriented and performance based

lymphatic drainage massage techniques, anatomy and physiology, and the underpinning knowledge of the lymphatic system and its components, in most states only licensed massage therapists with advanced training may perform this modality. Those aestheticians with advanced training are also permitted to perform this procedure, depending on the state licensure requirements.

Masks

Masks contain active ingredients in high concentrations. They are normally applied as the next-to-last step of a facial treatment. Masks intensify the treatment and work on the principles of occlusion.

There are three standard types of masks:

Gel-based masks can be used by all skin types and are very hydrating. Their gel form increases the moisture content of the skin.

Cream-based masks are nondrying, usually have calming and hydrating properties, and typically contain water soluble ingredients as the main components.

Clay masks are drying by nature and draw out impurities. They offer balancing and tightening. Manufacturers may design their clay masks to be setting (drying) or nonsetting types.

masks
high active ingredients in gel or cream form normally applied in the final step of a facial

Aestheticians are increasingly recognizing the benefits of adding in specialty masks such as layered masks, which involve layering the applications of serums, creams, and gel masks and finishing with a layer of a setting mask similar to plaster of Paris. Paraffin or thermal masks work from the premise of heat and are known for their benefits of penetrating specialty creams and ampoules. Freeze-dried collagen sheets have gained popularity and are similar to the freeze-dried collagen sheets obtained from a postmortem human donor used by plastic surgeons for lip implants. These sheets are absorbed into the body over a 6 to 12 month time period, and the patient's lips return to their original form. Aestheticians use free dried collagen sheets to offer surface hydration and to deliver specialty ingredients incorporated into the sheets targeted for specific skin types and conditions. These sheets are commonly used alone or in conjunction with ampoules for increased results.

back facials
facial treatments that involve cleansing, toning, exfoliating, masking, and massaging the back; they are similar to a standard facial and involve the same steps

▪ BACK FACIALS

Back facials are popular with acneic clients and women who are attending a special event where their dress reveals the shoulders and back. A back facial can be exfoliation oriented to reveal glowing skin or more clinically oriented, addressing conditions such as acne. Typically a back facial will achieve the same results as a standard facial. Some spas sell packages of back facials, typical to those for other types of facials, to clients who want to address sun damage or acne.

Back facials (see Figure 8–10) are an easy procedure to integrate into service menus as the equipment needed to provide one is similar to that of facials. Many back facials include the use of machines and steam. They follow the same protocols as a typical facial, with adjustments made for the skin type or condition.

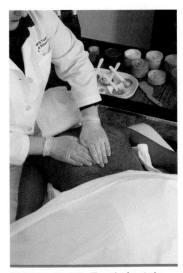

Figure 8–10 Back facials are popular with acneic clients and women who are attending an event where their dress reveals the shoulders and back

▪ FACIALS FOR MEN

In aesthetics, working with men can be quite different from working with women. Men can be very loyal customers. They make up 15 to 20 percent of the industry's clientele. The biggest challenge is to get a man to come in for the first time. Typically, once he sees the results, he will come back for more services. Offering special services designed just for men can be beneficial. Men prefer simple routines and multipurpose products with no fluff or fragrance. There are certain things to remember when performing a facial on a man. Massage and movement should be done in the same downward direction as the hair's growth. Sponges are preferable to cotton pads, which can catch on facial hair.

It is best to advise the client to avoid shaving immediately prior to coming in for a facial treatment as some exfoliation products on freshly shaven skin may be contraindicated. Folliculitis is commonly seen in men, especially those with coarse or wiry beards. Treatments for this include alleviating irritation, drying up and disinfecting pustules, and desensitizing the affected area as well as integrating high frequency into the facial for its antibacterial effects. Some facials may include the removal of ingrown hairs. A popular exfoliator to use in place of granules is enzyme peels as they are not difficult to remove on men with facial hair. They are also effective, as are AHAs, in assisting with pseudofollicular barbae.[13] When you provide treatments for men, you should consider a brand of home care that appeals to men. Men typically prefer very low maintenance, simple regimes and prefer tubes to pumps. In short, men like simplicity and are a relatively untapped market.

Conclusion

There are many types of facials, but all work around the standard seven steps of facials including: (1) cleansing, (2) analysis, (3) deep cleansing, exfoliation, extractions, (4) treat and correct, (5) massage, (6) mask, and (7) completion. There are many ways to vary the facials you offer your clients. With the advancement of new technologies, there are many new options available. Many aestheticians and spas are now recognizing that services and products specifically geared to men are a relatively untapped market and are becoming more and more in demand. Aestheticians are becoming more aware of the benefits of adding on services to their facials and integrating advanced technologies. The consumer is also becoming more educated, and the market is moving toward clinical facials. It is becoming easier for aestheticians to deliver results oriented skin care treatments, but, with this advancement in technology, there must also be an increase in the education needed. Many states are moving toward increasing the number of hours required to become a licensed aesthetician. States such as Utah and Virginia have a two-tiered approach, with a basic aesthetician who can perform spa related services and a master level aesthetician who is allowed to perform advanced modalities such as chemical exfoliation, microdermabrasion, and lymphatic drainage.

> > > **TOP 10 TIPS TO TAKE TO THE CLINIC**

1. Offer a variety of facials to address all skin types.
2. Educate the reception staff on the basic facts on the treatments you offer.
3. Do not overcrowd your menu and simplify descriptions.
4. Run monthly promotions highlighting different treatments.
5. Include men's facials on your menu.
6. Offer simple home-care protocols for men.
7. Design easy to follow home-care sheets to help clients maintain their treatment results.
8. Attend workshops and conferences to learn about new technology
9. Set goals for continuing education.
10. Do not be afraid to try new types of facials.

CHAPTER QUESTIONS

1. Name the seven steps to a facial.
2. Why is setup important?
3. What is the difference in a machine versus a manual facial?
4. Name some common aromatherapy oils used in skin care.
5. Name two types of facials that would benefit dehydrated clients.
6. Why would you not use paraffin on acneic clients?
7. Name the three types of standard masks.
8. How is a back facial similar to a regular facial?
9. How might a man's facial be different from a woman's facial?

CHAPTER REFERENCES

1. Worwood, V. (2001). *Aromatherapy for Beauty Therapist*. Clifton Park, NY: Thomson Delmar Learning.
2. D'Angelo, J., Dean, P., Deitz, S., Hinds, C., Lees, M., Miller, E., et al. (2003). *Milady's Standard: Comprehensive Training for Estheticians*. Clifton Park, NY: Thomson Delmar Learning.
3. http://www.catalystmagazine.net

4. *Fitzpatrick Skin Typing Chart (part 1—Genetic Disposition)*. Used with permission of the Medical Procedure Center, P.C., and adapted from multiple sources.
5. *Fitzpatrick Skin Typing Chart (part 2—Reaction to Sun Exposure)*. Used with permission of the Medical Procedure Center, P.C., and adapted from multiple sources.
6. *Fitzpatrick Skin Typing Chart (part 3—Tanning Habits)*. Used with permission of the Medical Procedure Center, P.C., and adapted from multiple sources.
7. *Fitzpatrick Skin Typing Chart (part 4—Scoring)*. Used with permission of the Medical Procedure Center, P.C., and adapted from multiple sources.
8. *Fitzpatrick Skin Typing Chart (part 5—Your Fitzpatrick Skin Type)*. Used with permission of the Medical Procedure Center, P.C., and adapted from multiple sources.
9. Rubin, M., MD. (1995). *Manual of chemical peels: Superficial and medium depth*. Philadelphia, PA: Lippincott Williams & Wilkins.
10. http://www.mayoclinic.com
11. Bitter, Patrick H. (2000). Noninvasive rejuvenation of photo-damaged skin using serial, full-face intense pulsed light treatments. *Dermatologic Surgery, 26,* 835.
12. http://www.vanderbilt.edu
13. D'Angelo, J., Dean, P., Deitz, S., Hinds, C., Lees, M., Miller, E., et al. (2003). *Milady's Standard: Comprehensive Training for Estheticians*. Clifton Park, NY: Thomson Delmar Learning.

BIBLIOGRAPHY

APA Optics, Inc. (2004, March 18). *Personal UV monitor*. Available at http://www.apaoptics.com

Bitter, Patrick H. (2000). Noninvasive rejuvenation of photodamaged skin using serial, full-face intense pulsed light treatments. *Dermatologic Surgery, 26,* 835.

D'Angelo, J., Dean, P., Deitz, S., Hinds, C., Lees, M., Miller, E., et al. (2003). *Milady's Standard: Comprehensive Training for Estheticians*. Clifton Park, NY: Thomson Delmar Learning

Deitz, S. (2004). *Milady's the Clinical Aesthetician*. Clifton Park, NY: Thomson Delmar Learning.

Genetree. (2004, February 28). *Genetree eye color inheritance chart*. Available at http://www.genetree.com

http://www.biotone.com

http://www.catalystmagazine.net

http://education.yahoo.com

http://www.mayoclinic.com

http://www.vanderbilt.edu

Institute for Medicine, Physics, and Biophysics. (2004, February 27). *Definitions (Working Group UVR)*. Available at http://i115srv. uv-wein.ac.at

The Lasky Clinic. (2004, March 1). *Mark Rubin, M.D.* Available at http://www.laskyclinic.com

Martini, F. H., Ober, W. C., Garrison, C. W., Welsh, K., Hutchings, R. T., et al. (2006). *Fundamentals of anatomy and physiology*. San Francisco, CA: Pearson Education.

MGH Hotline. (2003, August 22). *In memoriam: Thomas B. Fitzpatrick, MD, PhD*. Available at http://www.mgh.harvard.edu

Parks, J., MD, & Pierce, M., PA. (2002, May). *Effectively treating ethnic skin*. Available at http://www.skinandaging.com

Rubin, M., MD. (1995). *Manual of chemical peels: Superficial and medium depth*. Philadelphia, PA: Lippincott, Williams & Wilkins.

San Francisco Dermatology. (March 1, 2004). *Richard Glogau, MD*. Available at http://www.sfderm.com

Science Education Partnership. (2004, February 28). *The genetics of human eye color*. Available at http://www.seps.org

Thomas, C. L., MD, MPH (Ed.). (1997). *Taber's Cyclopedic Medical Dictionary* (Vol. 18). Philadelphia, PA: F. A. Davis Company.

Worwood, V. (2001). *Aromatherapy for Beauty Therapist*. Clifton Park, NY: Thomson Delmar Learning.

Marketing Your Spa Business

CHAPTER 9

KEY TERMS

acupressure

acupuncture

auriculotherapy

cost to acquire

cross-selling

database

ear reflexology

foot reflexology

hand reflexology

marketplace

powering the client
database

referral programs

understanding your
client

understanding your
competition

LEARNING OBJECTIVES

After completing this chapter, you should be able to:

1. Define in-house marketing strategies.

2. Identify how one can use in-house marketing strategies for a spa business.

3. Explain how appealing to the senses will be desirable to new and existing clients.

4. Identify some of the ways to enhance or expand existing treatments.

5. Explain some ways to use outside advertising as a means of marketing a spa business.

INTRODUCTION

Marketing your spa business, or any business, is vital to its long term success. When people think of marketing, they usually think of ads in newspapers or commercials on radio or television. These are indeed marketing devices, but they are not the most important, nor even the ones that will keep your clients coming back.

In an image business like the spa industry, certain aesthetic standards are desired by—even demanded by—a fickle clientele. Starting a spa is one thing, but keeping the clients coming back is an entirely different endeavor. Important goals are to keep existing clients returning for more treatments and to have them give referrals to their friends and colleagues. Achieving these goals will ensure the success of your spa business.

Aside from having a well-trained staff, a viable menu of treatment options, and a solid business plan, you will need to have an aesthetically pleasing environment in which to perform your treatments. The first impression the client has upon entering your business should be of a pleasant, clean facility. The best in-house marketing strategy you can have is to keep the client saying "wow" from the moment he or she walks in until the moment he or she leaves. A dazzled client will surely tell a friend of his or her experience. Conversely, a disappointed client will do the same.

■ IN-HOUSE MARKETING

In-house marketing is any marketing device that is used on the premises of your business to entice the client back to your business for future spa treatments. In-house strategies are among the most effective and the lowest cost means of attracting new clients and increasing revenue. By implementing cross-selling, **powering the client database**, and using **referral programs**, you can create a sophisticated, layered initiative to generate additional revenue as well as flex your know-how.

First, learn and implement **cross-selling**. This is a tactic that will begin to build your practice immediately. Cross-selling is the technique of taking a client who is active in one category and expanding her treatments into other categories. For example, a client getting a facial may also be a candidate for an opportunity to experience a body treatment. Cross-sales can be made in a couple of ways: first offer a gift certificate, followed by a discount on a package sale. Also, cross-selling can happen subtly when you combine procedures in a package. For example, when a client buys a facial package, include a couple of body treatments. Almost every-

powering the client database
in-house marketing strategy that involves innovative and detailed use of information already contained in a business database in order to increase traffic

referral programs
in-house marketing strategy that rewards an existing client for referring a new one

cross-selling
the process of selling related, peripheral items to a customer

one can benefit from the treatments provided in the spa, so it is really a win-win proposition for everyone.

Powering the database utilizes your existing database to uncover potential candidates for spa. This requires investigative work on the part of the staff, but it is worth it. It can cost 10 times more money to gain a new client than to keep an old client,[1] so get to work on those clients you already have in your database. Look through the database and find out who has not been into the facility for awhile. Evaluate the number of "lost clients" and create a cross-selling campaign to grab them back into the facility.

Creating new clients from your current database may seem redundant, but the use of a referral program will do a great job to create new clients. Most facilities experience at least a 30 percent referral rate. In other words, each month 30 percent of your new clients come from the referral of happy clients. Do you reward those clients who send you business? If not, why not? It is the easiest new client you will get, and she is presold because her friend told her that your facility was the best. Create a referral program for your established clients. Use gift certificates or cash rewards. Everybody wins.

Another essential means of in-house marketing is to provide literature describing the procedures the spa offers. Original literature specific to your spa can be informational, educational, and identifiable. If you do not print original literature, be sure to have literature that is supplied by product manufacturers, for example. If the manufacturer does not supply literature or brochures, several vendors create "boilerplate" literature that will work just fine. The important thing is that the literature be accurate and available. Included in the literature category should be "posttreatment" instructions. Even if these instructions are printed on your copy machine, you can still customize and dress up the presentation. However, the content is what is important, and function should take obvious precedence over form. Written posttreatment instructions are important to ensure the client follows your instructions and that there are not any misunderstandings.

> The best and worst forms of advertising are word of mouth or experience based. They are reliable, affordable, achievable, and manageable. Try to make each client satisfied enough to want to tell at least one other person. Just think of the profound effect this would have on your business success.

Maintaining a Zen-like Quality

Spa zen alludes to a relaxing state that is achieved through a combination of treatments and atmosphere. (See Figure 9–1.) Atmosphere is very important to the success of any business, as it is instrumental in attracting and keeping clientele. Atmosphere can be created through décor, music, aromatherapy, and even the staff's attitude (the amount of professionalism they exhibit, skill level, etc.). In order to be effective, atmosphere must be well planned and rehearsed. It must also be part of the entire staff's core belief at all times.

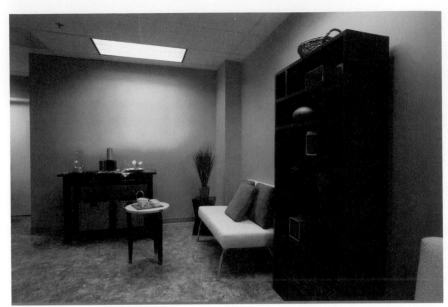

Figure 9–1 In order to be effective, atmosphere must be well planned and rehearsed. A relaxation room is a good place to start.

The overall impression a client receives when entering a spa has a great bearing on the effect the treatments will have on him or her. The ultimate outcome is that you want the clients to feel better leaving the spa than they did when they arrived. Since body treatments are about relaxation and rejuvenation, it is important that the spa itself conveys this. The best way to accomplish this is to consider the five senses and appeal to them individually.

Appealing to Sight

The first impression that anyone will have of your spa will be the way it looks. Different types of spas will have different types of design schemes. In fact, the type of spa ought to be the first consideration when establishing your design scheme. Whatever that scheme is, it should be visually pleasing. This means avoiding the extremes and realizing that having too much going on will be distracting. Similarly, high concept modern designs can seem cold and intimidating.

Appealing to sight does not just pertain to the physical environment, but also the aestheticians themselves. Appearances ought to be well maintained and put together. An aesthetician who looks neat and well groomed will inspire confidence and comfort on the part of the client.

Appealing to Smell

Aromatherapy can be used in the spa during facials, massages, and body treatments, as these services incorporate essential oils for various

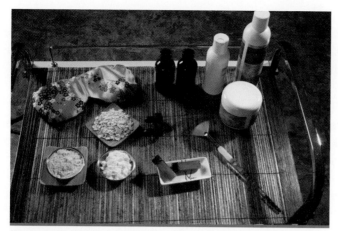

Figure 9–2 Aromatherapy can be used in the spa during facials, massages, and body treatments. These products add to the relaxation and environment of the spa and treatment.

therapeutic benefits. (See Figure 9–2.) The first place to use aromatherapy is in the reception area. Here aromatherapy mists can be used in the air to create a relaxing and soothing atmosphere for clients as they enter the spa.

Aromatic diffusers that plug into the wall are also ideal, as essential oil drops can be added to them to help create spa ambience. Other effective ways to use aromatherapy include adding a scent to linens or towels, dispersing the aroma into the air during the treatments, or performing a scalp massage with aromatic oils. Hydrotherapy is also an excellent opportunity to integrate aromatherapy into a treatment. Certain aromatherapy essential oils are quite effective for creating soothing baths, relaxing muscles, easing joints, or addressing skin conditions. Placing a few drops of lavender in the water and then soaking for 30 minutes in the tub while meditating, listening to tranquil music, or just relaxing has great stress relieving benefits. The most common method of applying essential oils is by massaging the diluted oils onto the body during a facial, body treatment, or massage. The essential oil is always mixed with carrier oil; it is never applied directly to the body. When using essential oils, be very aware of the contraindications and the client's health history.

Appealing to Sound

Sound is a very important component to spa ambiance. When people think of sound, the first thing they think about is music. Music is a valuable part of the spa experience. Music should be soothing with few or no words. Volume is also a consideration. Make sure that it is loud enough to hear, but not so loud that it is distracting.

Also associated with sound is tone of voice. Using a calm confident tone of voice will go far in enhancing the experience and establishing rapport with the client. Avoid using loud or condescending tones that will annoy clients.

Appealing to Touch

Touch is the most important sense in the spa setting. From the moment you shake hands with your client, your touch will drive the spa experience for the client. Whether giving a body treatment or a massage, your touch is necessary to the outcome. Tension, fear, and anxiety can all be conveyed through your touch, so it is important to have proper channels to manage stress and avoid passing the negativity to clients.

Appealing to Taste

Appealing to taste in a spa setting may not seem to jive, but doing so can have a great benefit to the client as well as the aesthetician. Having cold beverages, water in particular, will calm the client. Additionally, water will relieve water retention, maximizing many treatments performed at a spa. (See Figure 9–3.)

Enhancing or Expanding Treatment Options

Enhancing or expanding your treatment menu serves as a great excuse to advertise and provides an opportunity to keep up with the times. In the aesthetics industry, there are often new and innovative treatments that come in and out of fashion. While it not only serves you well to keep up with trends, having the savvy to know which ones appeal to your clientele will ensure your clients keep returning to your place of business.

Some of the services that you may want to consider adding to your menu list may stand alone or be used in conjunction with other treatments, for example, combining a relaxing facial with a massage treatment. That said, many spas have a signature treatment; something that they are known for and do "the best." Advertising your signature treatment and creating a package around that treatment is a smart business move. Some spas take the idea of a signature treatment one step further and create a signature treatment by age group or skin condition. (See Table 9–1.) This helps to further expand the client population and attract clients who otherwise might not have been interested in an average, everyday service.

Customizing Facials

One of the best ways to enhance an existing treatment is to customize a facial treatment. This can be done in conjunction with holidays, or on

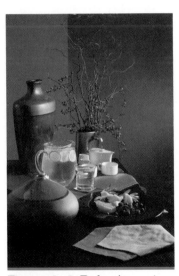

Figure 9–3 Refreshments should be offered in the relaxation room and after treatments

Table 9–1	Signature Treatments by Age Group
Age Group	**Possible Signature Treatments**
Teens	Facials directed at oily/acne skin
20s	Facials directed at acne skin
30s	Facials directed at the beginning signs of solar damage
40s	Facials directed at solar damage and the beginning signs of aging
50s	Facials directed at aging and premenopausal skin
60s	Facials for dry skin
70+	Facials for dry, thin skin

another rotating basis. For example, one might offer a pumpkin facial for autumn or Thanksgiving, or a chocolate facial for Valentine's Day or the client's birthday. The degree to which you switch the custom facials is an in-house decision based on the needs and responses of your clientele.

Massage

As mentioned above, adding a massage treatment to an existing treatment, or adding it as a stand-alone treatment, is a great way of expanding your business and enhancing the overall spa experience for your clients. Since the requirements for massage treatments vary from state to state, be sure to check licensure requirements in the state where you intend to practice, and limit the practice of massage treatments to individuals who are properly certified. In most spas, having an individual who is cross-trained in aesthetics and massage therapy is very desirable. (See Figure 9–4.)

Reflexology

Reflexology is a natural healing art, based on the principle that there are reflexes in the feet and hands that correspond to every part of the body. By stimulating and applying pressure to the feet or hands, you can increase circulation and promote specific bodily and muscular functions. Indeed, the feet and hands are more sensitive than most people realize. Similar to how we use our eyes to detect light, the hands and feet detect pressure, stretch, movement, and weight distribution. This in turn affects how the entire body carries itself.

As with massage, reflexology is a mechanical means of achieving relaxation. It is an ideal means of helping a client achieve a relaxed state while receiving a facial or another body treatment.

Developing packages of treatments, especially facials, is a smart business decision. Typically packages are designed to save the client money by a prepay discount and improve retention by increasing the number of times a client returns. The newest trend in packages is to combine different treatments to customize a package that meets the needs of the individual client, for example, facials combined with LED light treatments or even a massage. This kind of package exposes the client to several services and different clinicians. Furthermore, it should provide him or her with an improved result if the package is developed with his or her particular skin problem in mind.

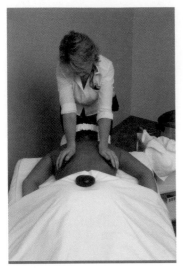

Figure 9–4 Massage is a good addition to the spa services

Reflexology can relieve energy blockages in the feet, hands, and even ears. Once the blockages are relieved, the corresponding body part is also likely to experience some form of relief. In general terms, the benefits of reflexology include the reduction of stress. Because the feet and hands help set the tension level for the rest of the body, they are an easy way to interrupt the stress signal and reset homeostasis, the body's equilibrium.[2] Reiki is a type of reflexology that emphasizes balancing the body's homeostatic equilibrium. Pressure points are chosen that realign the body's internal equilibrium, resulting in smoother body function. It is thought that this type of reflexology improves digestion, relieves stress pattern fat deposits, and improves energy levels.

One of the foremost benefits of reflexology is the energy restorative benefits. Many practitioners of reflexology believe that energy healing can assist with a wide variety of physical, mental, and emotional ailments because it works with the body's natural capacity for self-healing. The power of energy healing comes from the early identification of disruptions and disturbances at the level of energy before they manifest in diseases and disorders. It is believed that this energy gives advance notice of problems, as well as precious time to heal issues before they become serious illnesses.[3]

Foot reflexology (see Figure 9–5) is the theory that all organs and glands are represented through the feet. It is believed that a reflexology

foot reflexology
an ancient Chinese technique that uses pressure-point massage on the feet to restore the flow of energy throughout the entire body

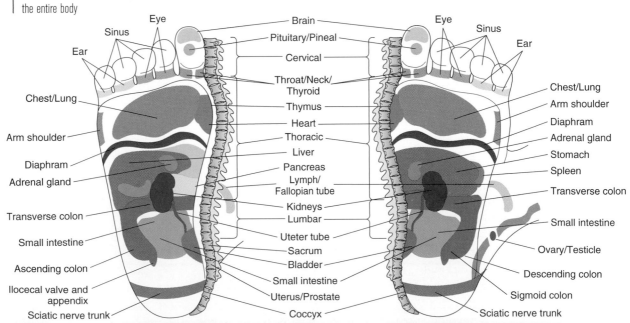

Figure 9–5 Reflexology is a natural healing art

foot massage can have healing effects on other parts of the body. Recognized benefits from receiving a foot reflexology treatment include increased circulation, relaxation, and release of tensions.

Reflexology pressure, which resembles something similar to the movement of an inchworm,[4] can be applied to reflex points in a variety of ways. The fingers and thumbs are commonly used to reflex areas of the feet and hands.

Hand reflexology (see Figure 9–6), while not as well known as foot reflexology, is equally as effective in balancing the body, improving nerve and blood supply, and relieving stress and tension. The hands are not as sensitive as the feet and the reflexes are much deeper. As with the feet, there are reflexes on the hand that relate to all organs, glands, and parts of the body. A reflexologist can produce these positive health benefits for clients by stimulating hand reflexes using special thumb and finger techniques.[5] Once an individual is properly trained in reflexology, he or she can add this service to almost any treatment.

According to the principles of **ear reflexology** or auricular therapy, each area of the ear corresponds to a different anatomical portion of the body. Stimulation of these ear points over time exerts certain therapeutic effects on those parts of the body with which they are associated.

> In research studies, reflexology has proven effective in providing relief for over 60 disorders ranging from heart disease to epilepsy.

hand reflexology
an ancient Chinese technique that uses pressure-point massage on the hands to restore the flow of energy throughout the entire body

ear reflexology
an ancient Chinese technique that uses pressure-point techniques on the ears to restore the flow of energy throughout the entire body

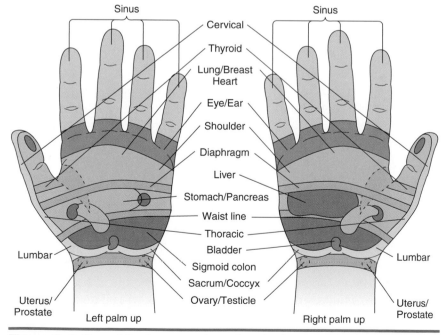

Sinus   Sinus
Cervical
Thyroid
Lung/Breast Heart
Eye/Ear
Shoulder
Diaphragm
Liver
Stomach/Pancreas
Waist line
Thoracic
Bladder
Lumbar   Lumbar
Sigmoid colon
Sacrum/Coccyx
Uterus/Prostate   Ovary/Testicle   Uterus/Prostate
Left palm up   Right palm up

Figure 9–6 One of the foremost benefits of reflexology is the energy

auriculotherapy

also known as auricular therapy (ear acupuncture), this is a form of alternative medicine based on the idea that the ear is a microsystem, meaning that the entire body is represented on the auricle (or auricula, or pinna—the outer portion of the ear) in a similar fashion to reflexology (zone therapy) and iridology (iridodiagnosis), and that the entire body can be treated by stimulation of the surface of the ear exclusively

acupressure

an ancient healing therapy, originating in Asia over 5,000 years ago, that utilizes the fingers to depress key locations on the skin's surface to prompt healing within the body

acupuncture

treatment that involves penetrating the skin with thin, solid, metallic needles that are manipulated by the hands or by an electrical stimulation to prompt healing within the body

Paul Nogier, MD, a French neurosurgeon, is honored as the father of **auriculotherapy**. The map he created describes the ear as an upside down fetus with the lower ear representing parts on the upper body, while the upper ear represents parts of the lower body.

It has been reported that it is possible to diagnose a variety of pathological conditions by examining the ear. Reflexologists use specific touch techniques applied to the outer ear to help different parts of the body relax so that all of its parts function better, thus helping the body to better heal itself.[6]

Acupressure and Acupuncture

Acupressure, an ancient healing therapy that originated in Asia over 5,000 years ago, utilizes the fingers to depress key locations on the skin's surface to prompt healing within the body. Acupressure is similar to acupuncture and uses the same reference points on the body. It is commonly used to promote stress reduction and alleviate acute and chronic conditions.[7]

There are two popular methods of acupressure application, which vary only by their degree of pressure. Shiatsu acupressure uses vigorous and firm pressure application. Jin Shin acupressure uses a gentler form, holding the points for a moment or two. A typical acupressure session is done in a relaxing environment and does not require the removal of clothing.

Acupuncture focuses on a holistic, energy-based approach to the individual, rather than a disease-oriented diagnostic (see Table 9–2) and treatment model. The acupuncture treatment involves penetrating the skin with thin, solid, metallic needles that are manipulated by the hands or by electrical stimulation.

The general theory of acupuncture (see Figure 9–7) is based on the premise that there are patterns of energy flow through the body that are essential for good health. Disruptions of this flow are believed to be responsible for disease. The acupuncturist can correct imbalances of flow at identifiable points close to the skin.[8]

Becoming qualified to perform acupuncture is not as easy as it may seem. Acupuncture is a difficult practice to master because of the use of the needles and the complexity of the mapping of areas specific to treatment. Further complicating matters is the varying degrees of regulation from one state to the next. Currently, 44 states regulate the practice of acupuncture, while six do not. Rules in the 44 states that do regulate the practice are somewhat variant. Before considering adding this service to your menu, be sure you are familiar with the statutes in your state of practice.

Table 9–2   Conditions Acupuncture Might Treat

Acne	Gum disease
Addiction	Hay fever
AIDS	Headache
Allergies	Heartburn
Alzheimer's	Hemorrhoids
Angina	Hypertension
Anxiety	Impotence
Arthritis	Indigestion
Asthma	Infertility
Back pain (self-help)	Irritable bowel syndrome
Back pain (Chinese medicine)	Insomnia
Benign prostatic hyperplasia	Kidney stones
Breast cancer	Lung cancer
Breast lumps	Male infertility
Cancer	Memory loss
Candidiasis (yeast infection)	Meniere's disease
Carpal tunnel syndrome	Menopause
Cholesterol, high	Menstrual cramps
Chronic fatigue syndrome	Muscle strain and sprain
Constipation	Osteoporosis
Crohn's disease	Parkinson's disease
Depression	Premenstrual syndrome
Dermatitis (eczema)	Preventative medicine
Diabetes	Psoriasis
Diarrhea	Rheumatoid arthritis
Diverticular disease	SARS
Endometriosis	Shingles
Eye diseases	Sinusitis

(Continued)

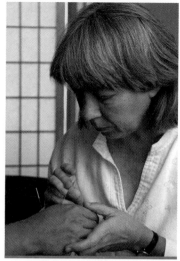

Figure 9–7 Acupressure is an ancient healing therapy that originated in Asia over 5,000 years ago

Table 9–2 Conditions Acupuncture Might Treat—cont'd	
Female sexual dysfunction	Stroke
Fibroids	Tinnitus
Fibromyalgia	Trigeminal neuralgia
Flu (and colds)	Ulcerative colitis
Glaucoma	Urinary incontinence
Gout	Urinary tract infection

Keeping Your Business Moving

In order for your new spa service to thrive, you will need to keep up with the trends, regulations, and competition associated with your new service, or even the spa industry at large. These are collectively referred to as your business landscape. The business landscape will be the deciding factor in many areas, most notably, marketing your spa program accurately and effectively.

Three deeply intertwined aspects of evaluating your business landscape are the marketplace, clients, and competition. Independently and consequentially, these three components are in a state of constant change. By identifying the present conditions of each, you have defined the current landscape. The **marketplace** is different in every city, and it is sometimes even more localized than your city—it may be your local community. Therefore, in order to have a firm grasp on the marketplace, you must understand your city and local community.

With a comprehensive understanding of local dynamics, narrowing the general population down to your business's client base is the second and most misunderstood component of the business landscape. **Understanding your client** will have a domino effect on marketing, pricing, and many other components that are critical to the success of your business.

Finally, while knowing your marketplace and your clients will have a significant role in your daily operations, **understanding your competition** does not. Therefore, it should not have an equal share of consideration. Worrying about your competition could become a distraction (or an obsession) that will only harm your business. You should limit your understanding of competition to the few bits of information you really need to compile about your competition (prices, menu, and promotions).

In addition to keeping current with your business landscape, moving forward includes accurate and regular monitoring and daily tracking of

marketplace
any environment where two or more people buy or sell a product or service

understanding your client
component of the business landscape during which a business evaluates and acquaints itself with its target demographics

understanding your competition
component of the business landscape during which a business evaluates its competition in terms of pricing, procedures, demographics, and promotions

operations and business risks. Establishing indicators and goals and understanding your financial statements plays a pivotal role. Most important are indicators and goals. Review indicators and goals weekly to evaluate the performance of the facility and the aesthetician. This review will pave the road to your success. In the following sections, we discuss the issues of your business landscape in more detail.

Understanding the Client

Understanding your client is helpful when designing your marketing plan. Most marketing principles are general and are considered "the norm" because they have proven to change or modify consumer behavior. However, with a well-thought interpretation of your potential clients you will be able to tailor your campaign to your client base, as opposed to broader populations. Enhanced collection and analysis will help you refine your campaign from conception to implementation. This will include the analysis of the demographic of the current database and what secrets might be buried that will assist you with a deeper understanding of the client.

An analysis of the existing client base will give you a composite sketch of your target demographic. The information you should seek includes service preferences, price sensitivity, age, household income, knowledge of the industry, referral source, and preconceived notions of the facility and services.

Take note of the existing clients in the current **database** who might be interested in the new services you plan to offer based upon your composite sketch criteria. This can be done two ways—through a survey or by a mathematical analysis based on growth. If you use a survey, the process is very simple. Create a survey that clients can fill out while waiting for their treatment. Filling out the questionnaire can include a spa treatment offer at an "introductory promotional price." Those who are not in the facility during the time you are doing the survey can be called or emailed with the survey.

Using the mathematical approach may not be as insightful but is still effective. Knowing the number of clients you currently have in your database, realistically project the potential number of clients that will cross over to spa. Keep the number low, for example, 2 to 5 percent of the database.

With this information in hand, create an in-house campaign to capture these clients to the new treatment. Current clients should be the first to experience the treatment and enjoy your new menu offerings. To further increase the number of clients, create a referral offer for those who experience the treatment and refer a friend.

database
an electronic compilation of extensive categorical information relevant to business processes, such as marketing or inventory

Understanding the Competition

Your competition is everywhere, even outside your business sector. Like it or not, the ideal is the marker against which the commonplace is compared. Your waiting area will be compared to the most exquisite furnishing fit for royalty. Your customer service will be held up to virtually unattainable standards. And, yes, your treatment programs will be expected to surpass the results of the leading plastic surgeons. This is just the way the client thinks. Other spas across town and the Fortune 500 conglomerates across the globe are all your competition, but you must shrink your description of the competition down to a bulleted list of information, which can facilitate your individual business goals. This does not suggest that you put undeserving emphasis on "keeping up with the Joneses" or overreaching your own business goals; rather your business success will be served best by an internal motivation to satisfy your own clients.

The competition across town or across the hallway can be distracting. You want to know what they are doing, who their clients are, and what their treatments are. It is important to know what your competition is doing, but do not be obsessed with them. The few key points that you should know about your competition are their pricing, common procedures, demographic target, and promotions. Once you know these things or have an idea of the direction of their business, stay informed but leave it alone. Use your time efficiently, by growing your own business and not paying attention to someone else's.

> Competition across the country is important because it gives you an idea of the direction of the industry. Look for a couple of very progressive businesses on each coast and in the middle of the country. Stay on top of what they are doing, including their pricing, procedures, promotions, literature and written materials, and Web site promotions. This will help you to know the trends and fads that are developing in the industry and adjust your business if you wish.

■ OUTSIDE MARKETING

Creating marketing strategies and watching them "bring in the clients" can be very rewarding at times, and equally disconcerting at other times. Business growth followed by success is dependent on innovative and effective marketing. The marketing plan you create should utilize as many tactics as possible, as each of them will have a different reach, appeal, and anticipated impact on the business. These tactics should include direct mail, email, newspaper, radio, in-house strategies, and literature to mention a few. (See Table 9–3.)

Direct Mail

Direct mail is commonly used to introduce new services. The spa usually sends out a card or letter with an offer attached. Direct mail has a success rate of 1.5 percent or less. The average facility may believe this to be a

Table 9–3   Marketing Strategies

Marketing Strategy	Breadth of Market Reach	Cost	Cost to Acquire Risk
Direct mail	Low	High	High
Email	Low	Low	Low
Newspaper	Moderate	High	High
Billboard	Moderate	Moderate	Moderate
Radio commercials	Moderate	Low	Low
Regional magazine	High	High	Moderate
Local affiliate television commercials	High	High	Moderate

terrific way to introduce a service or product, but it can be expensive, not to mention that it is often considered junk mail and immediately tossed in the trash. Let us take a look.

If you send out 1,000 cards you will get, at best, 15 clients through the door. If the direct mail piece cost $2.00 per card plus postage, the total per card is $2.41. The total cost for the mailer will be $2,410.00. That means each of the 15 clients who come through the door must spend $158.00 to cover just the direct cost of the mailer. In other words, that is before you begin to cover the overhead or make any money. An unexpectedly low yield could end up being very costly. While you can be successful (success depends on the match of potential client to service) with direct mail, as well as all strategies, do the math to make sure the ends justify the means. Bearing in mind that direct mailings have unpredictable outcomes, consider taking proactive steps to decrease the risk by trimming the fat from your mailing pool. Send direct mail pieces to only those clients who have responded positively to an in-house survey or who have been into the facility in the past six months. Also, those clients who have responded to a mailer before are likely to respond again. In addition, consider a "cross-selling" direct mail campaign that combines one treatment, for example, Restylane or Botox, with a promotional spa treatment. Because of the unpredictable nature of direct mailings, mail the offer to a selected number of more qualified clients rather than your entire database.

Email

It is to your advantage to make it easy and rewarding for your existing clients to volunteer their email addresses for in-house marketing and promotional use. By far, email is the most cost effective means of communicating with your clients. You can develop regular email specials and introduce new offerings with little effort and surprising results. When you put promotional signs in your office that say "Ask about our email-only specials" you will be surprised how many people will give you their email addresses, because no one wants to be left out when there is a special available. While email can be challenging from the perspective of aged email addresses and the possibility of your messages getting caught in spam, it is still worth doing—remember it is virtually free.

Newspaper

Newspaper advertising is tried and true. In most cities every weekend there are literally hundreds of ads for plastic surgery, spas, and medical skin care. Is your ad special? Or is it just one in the maze of many? Are you participating in "advertorials" or inserting a special tear-out newsletter? What is the competition right next to you doing? Newspapers can be an expensive tactic for acquiring new clients. The question that must be answered when it comes to newspaper advertising (as with all tactics) is the **cost to acquire**. In other words how much money must be spent to get one new client to walk through the door? Taken one step further, how many appointments did it take for the client to spend enough money to cover the cost of the newspaper ad and begin to produce a profit for your facility? Add into the financial mix the variable costs of ad design and any additional marketing, and you may find that newspaper ads are pretty expensive unless you can really attract a number of clients.

cost to acquire
the average cost per new customer of any one marketing strategy

Radio

Radio advertising is a viable option for smaller markets. In larger metropolitan areas like Los Angeles or New York, the reach of the radio station may be too great to merit radio advertising. In other words, a large percentage of potential clients are simply too far away to consider driving to your facility. Even under this condition, radio will provide great name recognition and tremendous branding, but the important question to ask is, What is the objective of radio advertising? If it is to attract clients, the larger the size of the metropolis, the greater the risk of unsatisfactory new client yield. With this in mind, in smaller communities radio may work well, especially if there is an AM drive time slot and a DJ who will give a live advertisement or, better yet, a testimonial.

Conclusion

Any business knows that the key to a business's survival is effective marketing. Yet how you market your business is a tricky decision that is very specific to your business. Over time, you will find that you will need to evaluate the success of your marketing strategies, and they will need to be evaluated and adjusted. Knowing your demographic is vital to doing this. Keeping tabs on who you want to come to your spa, and who is actually coming to your spa, as well as knowing how they heard of you is essential. More important is to make certain that those who do come to your spa leave happy. These happy clients are your key to success. After all, no matter how much you advertise, no matter how clever your marketing strategy, if you do not make your clients happy, your marketing strategy, as well as your business, will fail.

▶ ⟩ ⟩ TOP 10 TIPS TO TAKE TO THE CLINIC

1. Maintaining an existing client is just as important, if not more so, than acquiring a new one.

2. In-house marketing is an important step to maintaining existing clients.

3. Word of mouth advertising is the best way to keep clients coming into your spa business.

4. Cross-selling and providing literature are great ways to entice existing clients to try newer or existing treatment options they had not yet considered.

5. The overall appearance of your spa and its treatment areas is just as important to marketing your spa as an effective advertising campaign.

6. Appealing to all of the client's senses is an effective step toward achieving client satisfaction.

7. Expanding or enhancing existing treatment options as well as adding new menu items is a good way to keep clients interested.

8. Understanding your clients, the competition, and the marketplace will keep your spa business competitive.

9. Using outside marketing will draw new clients into your spa business.

10. Your choice of outside marketing should be a careful decision based on your businesss demographics and goals.

CHAPTER QUESTIONS

1. What is the difference between in-house and outside marketing strategies?

2. Give examples of each.

3. Why is it important to maintain a client database?

4. Give two examples of cross-selling. Why is cross-selling a valuable tool?

5. What is the best advertising strategy?

6. Why is it important to maintain a "zen-like" quality in your spa business?

7. Identify some of the methods one might use to appeal to the clients' senses.

8. Why is it important to expand existing treatments? What about adding new ones?

9. Explain what reflexology is. Identify the different types.

10. What is the difference between acupuncture and acupressure?

11. What are the three most important things a spa manager or owner needs to know in order to keep a spa business running for the long term?

12. List some of the types of outside marketing one might consider. Explain the pros and cons of each.

CHAPTER REFERENCES

1. Keller, K. L., Sternthal, B., & Tybout, A. (2002). Three questions you need to ask about your brand. *Harvard Business Review, 80*(9).

2. Bauer, M. (2005). *Healing power of acupressure and acupuncture*. New York: Avery.

3. http://education.yahoo.com

4. http://www.auriculotherapy.co

5. http://www.energymedicinedirectory.com

6. http://www.acupuncture.com

7. Bek, L., & Pullar, P. (1994). *Healing with chakra energy: Restoring the natural harmony of the body*. Rochester, VT: Destiny Books.

8. Kluck, M. (2001). *Hands on feet: The new system that makes reflexology a snap*. Philadelphia, PA: Running Press Book Publishers.

BIBLIOGRAPHY

American Management Association. (2004, February 15). *A baker's dozen pricing strategies*. Available at http://www.amanet.org

Bauer, M. (2005). *Healing power of acupressure and acupuncture*. New York: Avery.

Beer, K., MD. (2003, September). *The cosmetic clinic: Six secrets to success.* Available at http://www.skinandaging.com

Bek, L., & Pullar, P. (1994). *Healing with chakra energy: Restoring the natural harmony of the body.* Rochester, VT: Destiny Books.

Bennis, W. G., & Thomas, R. J. (2002). The crucibles of leadership. *Harvard Business Review, 80*(9).

Canada Business Service Centre. (2004, February 15). *Setting the right price.* Available at http://www.cbsc.org

Cosmetic Surgery Times. (2001, August). *How to buy a spa system without getting skinned.* Available at http://www.cosmeticsurgerytimes.com

Entrepreneur.com. (2001, October 2). *Avoid these "destroy your business" pitfalls.* Available at http://www.entrepreneur.com

FaceForum. (2004, March 10). *Spa costs: How much does spa cost?* Available at http://www.faceforum.com

Gail, S. (2003, July 1). *Mirror, mirror on the wall, are men so vain after all?* Available at http://www.cosmeticsurgerytimes.com

Grima, D. (2004, February 15). *Keeping tabs on your competition.* Available at http://www.santuccibrown.com

http://education.yahoo.com

http://www.acupuncture.com

http://www.auriculotherapy.com

http://www.energymedicinedirectory.com

Intermediainc.com Weekend Reading. (2001, July 27). *Acquire consumers for show, retain customers for the dough.*

Keller, K. L., Sternthal, B., & Tybout, A. (2002). Three questions you need to ask about your brand. *Harvard Business Review, 80*(9).

Khurana, R. (2002). The curse of the superstar CEO. *Harvard Business Review, 80*(9).

Kluck, M. (2001). *Hands on feet: The new system that makes reflexology a snap.* Philadelphia, PA: Running Press Book Publishers.

MarketingTeacher.com. (2004, February 13). *Pricing strategies lesson.* Available at http://www.marketingteacher.com

Matarasso, S. L., Glogau, R.G., & Markley, A. C. (1994, June). Wood's Lamp for superficial chemical peels. *Journal of American Academic Dermatology, 30*(6), 988–992.

Millenium Research Group. (2002, July). *US spa market 2002.* Available at http://www.mindbranch.com

Nemko, M. (March, 2000). *Perfecting your pricing strategies.* Available at http://www.entrepreneur.com

Obagi. (2004, March 10). *Selecting a spa machine.* Available at http://www.obagi-me.com

Parisian Peel Medical Spa. (2004, March 10). *Spa skin renewal market study confirms growth, cites "second generation technology".* Available at http://www.parisianpeel.com

Parisian Peel Medical Spa. (2000, October 10). *Aesthetic buyers guide: Spa market study defines industry leaders and market size.* Available at http://www.parisianpeel.com

Smith-Isroelit, B. (2004, January 21). *Spa finder's 2004 trends and predictions.* Available at http://www.spatrade.com

Spatrade. (2004, February 5). *Spas leading outlets for professional skin care brands.* Available at http://www.spatrade.com

Troy, B. (2003, October 1). *Patient experience makes your bottom line.* Available at http://www.cosmeticsurgerytimes.com

Tutor2u.com. (2004, February 13). *Pricing.* Available at http://www.tutor2u.net

Urbany, J. (2003, Fall). *Getting the price right: What gets in the way.* Available at http://www.nd.edu

Wills, P. (1995). *The reflexology manual: An easy-to-use illustrated guide to the healing zones of the hands and feet.* Rochester, VT: Healing Arts Press.

The Business of Spa Treatments

CHAPTER 10

KEY TERMS

accounts payable

accounts receivable

annual business plan

balance sheet

clinic protocols

cost of goods sold

database

deferred revenue

direct costs

economy pricing

goals

income statement

indicator hot-sheet

indicators

indirect costs

inventory

overhead costs

penetration pricing

premium pricing

pricing strategies

product bundling pricing

professional ethics

purchasing

standard pricing policy

yearly business objectives

LEARNING OBJECTIVES

After completing this chapter, you should be able to:

1. Understand the business environment.
2. Learn about the components of a business plan.
3. Learn how to establish and evaluate goals and indicators.
4. Understand the components of cost analysis.
5. Define the direct and indirect costs.

INTRODUCTION

Writing a business plan may seem simple. Initially it is simply writing down your vision or dream of what you want the business to look like and expanding on the concept. This is the fun part, putting the dream on paper. But once this is accomplished, it is necessary to take the process to the next step. Undeniably, this written process will include information about operations and marketing and will identify the management team. It should also include all the financial details about how the spa will operate and ultimately be successful. Typically, writing a business plan will be wrought with details you usually do not think about, and it will take more time than you anticipated. That is the beauty of a business plan—it makes you *think* and *plan*. In the process of thinking about how you will develop your business, you will have to answer questions and solve initial problems. This process helps to make your plan solid and void of potential holes that could later cause problems. Spa treatments are a luxury to many people and consequently do not create an immediate need for repeat business. It is the challenge and responsibility of the spa director, marketing director, and aesthetician, as a team, to create the need for additional repeat visits. Repeating appointments is called retention, and those treatments that respond best to a monthly appointment, such as a facial, are extremely valuable to the clinician and spa alike. Processes to retain the clients should also be part of the business plan. And all of this is just to create a plan to start a business. Each year a successful business will rewrite the business plan along with the budget for the upcoming year.

The initial business plan will obviously be far more detailed and extensive than the ongoing plans that will be written each year. Our discussion will begin with the initial business plan: what is needed and how it should be structured.

GETTING YOUR BUSINESS STARTED

Getting your spa business started can be both exciting and challenging. But, as stated, it requires a plan. A business plan is like a road map; it guides you and shows you which direction to go. Without one you may not know where you are going, and this could be the difference between success and failure when important questions need to be answered. The table of contents of a primary business plan includes the following: the executive summary, the management team, the market, the spa model, operations, marketing, and the financial models. A business plan with this amount of detail will be accepted by your bank or other potential investors as a complete document for financing. It is a lot of work, but it will pay off in the near term when the spa opens and as it grows. As time goes on, you will not need a business plan of this detail. But each year as you develop your budget it is wise to update the business plan, especially in the marketing and operations categories.

The Executive Summary

The executive summary tells about the business and the objectives of the business plan. This section often will have a toned down version of your dream. It will also include information about the financing that is being sought. Other topics to be considered in the executive summary include a quick overview of the market, competition, and business strategy. These topics should dovetail to the experience of the management team. Each of the categories found in the executive summary will have an individual chapter in the business plan. Therefore, the objective of the executive

The Executive Summary

Overview of the Company
Include the reasons for anticipated success
History of the company

Management
A brief statement about the strength of the management team
A boxed feature with the names of the management team and their recent job histories

The Market
An introduction to the market that will build a foundation for the reader to be used in later sections
Strong statistics that you will be able to discuss

Marketing
A brief introduction to the most effective means of marketing, including information about the brand attributes of the company

Business Strategy
Four to five points of the basic business strategy that will make your company successful, including a brief statement about the growth or expansion strategy

Competition
An introduction to the competition in the marketplace

summary is to introduce the subject with top line information. The details of the subject matter will be found in the individual chapters.

The Management Team

The section that is titled "The Management Team" is just that: it talks about the team you have pulled together. Who will be the president, the secretary, and the treasurer? This section also explains who will be in director positions. For example, who will be the Director of Marketing of operations? Titles are not particularly important to some people, but titles create a sense of organization. As the business begins to take off, it is important that the staff understand who is in charge and what the hierarchy of the organization is. Once each individual is identified, a small biography of each person is necessary, a curriculum vitae (CV). The CV should include educational information as well as information about professional experiences that relate to the current venture. Furthermore, this section may expand into a detailed description of the company and its history.

Also include in this section information about the corporate structure and how the regulatory issues will be managed.

The Market

Before you even begin to write your plan, market research is required. Market research will involve many important topics, among them: how many spas are in the area, what types of spas they are, what treatments are provided, and how much they charge for those treatments. Furthermore, specific demographics should be included, such as the average client age and average household income. Other important market research would include what kinds of promotions might work or have been successful at other spas. All of this information should be written into the business plan. As you prepare this information, consider using graphs or pie charts. When communicating statistics, visuals convey information in a concise format, are easy on the eye, and break up the copy of a plan. Finally, if you are preparing this document for a bank or for venture money, it should include information about documented national trends.

Marketing

This category is usually everyone's favorite. It is great to watch clients come through the door. But without proper planning, hiring, training, and launching, there is no reason for marketing. Subjects that should be discussed in this section can be broken down into two categories: inside marketing and outside marketing. Inside marketing includes those tactics

The Management Team

President and CEO—This should include a CV or resume of this person in a written commentary, not in a traditional resume format. Integrated into the discussion of job history should be information about how the company was founded and why this person has been chosen to run the company. If this person is a founder or co-founder, this information should be included.

CFO or Chief Financial Officer—As for the president, this person should be identified by a job history. If he or she is a founder, it should be so noted. The CFO is extraordinarily important to those reviewing a business plan for financing. A strong person in this position will help to improve the odds for receiving financing.

COO or Chief Operating Officer—Initially this position may not be filled, especially if the founder is involved in the operations. If there is not a high level position such as this being filled, it should be noted whether a director position is to be filled such as Director of Operations. Once again, be sure to include the relevant job history.

Director of Marketing—Sometimes the marketing position is not considered an important role in the executive team. But, knowing how to drive business through the door and improve the spa's retention of clients is essential to the overall success. So if you have a marketing person in mind who has an impressive resume, be sure to include him or her in this section.

If there are other key persons on the executive management team who bring authority, be sure to include them in this section.

that one would use with the current clients. Examples of this might be holiday promotions, "bring a friend" promotions, or sales on products. Outside marketing includes those tactics that are focused on the public and directed at those individuals who are not currently your clients. Examples of outside marketing are seminars, Web sites, and coupons. All of the ideas for inside and outside marketing must be discussed in this section. It is a lot of work to compile these ideas. Furthermore, it should be estimated how much money it will require to get a client through the door. This is called the cost to acquire. Cost to acquire is an important concept because until you understand how much it will cost you to get a client you cannot really understand when you will begin to make money on the client. Once again, all of this should be shown in the business plan.

Business Strategy

This section is where you articulate your dream in detail. For example, this section should include information about your values and the value you intend to provide for your clients. How will you build customer relationships and create business alliances? All of the services that are offered will be listed in this section (use a table for clarity). This section will also include some information about who will provide the services and how the services are provided.

Operations should also be included in this section of the business plan. It will take a look at how the processes work, or, in other words, how a client is processed through the spa. This should also include information about the spa menu and the equipment that will be needed to accomplish these services. The rationale for providing these services should be included.

Competition

Competition is an important subject for everyone involved in the business. Break the information down into separate and meaningful categories such as competition and the day spa, competition and the medical spa, competition and the cosmetic market. Make the information easy to digest for the reader. A table might be helpful in this section.

Remember that any market information that you have gathered should have a source of information. It is good to footnote any statistics or market research that you have done for the business plan.

The Financial Model

The financial model is at the end of your business plan, but it is the section that anyone looking at your plan will be the most interested in. How will you make the money? How much money will you make? How fast will you become profitable? How much does it cost to acquire each new client? How fast does that individual client start sending money to the bottom line? In short, this is the section of the plan that determines whether or not your business idea is viable. It is also the section that will most likely determine whether or not you can get money to start your business.

The financial plan section of the business plan consists of several important documents: financial statements that include the projected income statement, a detailed cash flow projection, and the growth plan. All documents require a brief explanation or analysis. Furthermore, any actual financial performance or audit information that is relevant should be included.

ACQUIRING FINANCING

Once the business plan is complete, you are ready to search for financing. At this point the amount of money necessary to launch the business should be clear. The amounts should be articulated in the projected cash flow and growth plans.

Nothing can be more unnerving than looking for money. Typically, someone looking to finance his or her business is both excited and anxious. The execution of your dream is in the hands of someone who views it simply as a business venture, not a passion. As the founder, this can be a frustrating situation for you. Nevertheless, try to look at this process as dispassionately as possible. If you look at it as a business, then you will be viewed as a professional worth considering as a financial partnership.

There are two important pieces of advice to be considered when looking for start-up money. First, take the *best offer* for the business. Sometimes, the best offer may not have to do with money. Rather it will include the help you will get running the company or the contacts that will help you get to the next level of growth. This is especially true in the case of an angel investor. Next, believe in yourself. There will be more than one offer. Do not feel that you need to take the first offer that comes along. If it is not a good deal, keep looking. Do not give up half of your company to a venture opportunity because you are afraid it will be your only chance.

Finally, remember that there are many ways to finance your company. Among some of the ways to consider are bank loans, venture money, mezzanine financing, angel financing, SBA loans, family money or loans, partnerships, and self-financing. Choose to investigate several options to ensure that you have the best choice for your company.

BUYING EQUIPMENT

Because skin care is becoming "high tech," evaluating the equipment carefully and developing a spa menu accordingly will be important. High tech equipment will be necessary to maintain a competitive edge. Be sure to consider, however, whether the treatment will be a "here today gone tomorrow" fad or whether it has staying power. Think about the cost of the equipment and how many treatments will need to be done each month to cover this cost. However, do not forget it is not just the cost of the equipment that should be considered, it is also the cost of the employee, the training, and the overhead. But, we are getting a little ahead of ourselves. Let us start at the beginning.

Whether you are a new business owner who is on the threshold of an exciting new venture or part of a well established facility looking to upgrade to something new, **purchasing** the right equipment is crucial to your ultimate success. But, shopping for new equipment, whether it is a bed, an IPL machine, or a microdermabrasion machine, can be a challenge. While price is obviously important, it should not be the primary consideration. To ensure that you get a machine that fits your budget and meets your needs, begin by evaluating the features you are looking for rather than just the price.

When considering an equipment manufacturer, research to find out if the company is well established. Do they have reliable safety and performance records? Do they have a reputation for quality and service? Will the company be "here today and gone tomorrow"? If the company is new to the industry, have they made other devices with a solid reputation? Are they the primary manufacturer or a reseller? Will they stand behind their products and provide service and support? What type and duration of warranties are available? If you know someone from a facility that has been using a certain type of machine, ask his or her opinion. Usually you will get an unbiased assessment. Once the questions of the manufacturer are answered, the issues of the equipment itself can begin to be addressed. By evaluating certain features of the equipment, you will begin to hone in on the price you will need to pay to achieve your **goals**.

Depending on the piece of equipment you are looking at, your warranty should be one year with potential options for renewal. Be sure you get in writing the company's procedure for "down machines"—those that are broken or otherwise inoperable. Will the manufacturer or reseller provide a comparable loaner? How fast can they get the loaner to you? Will the loaner be free or will it be a rental? A broken machine without prompt service or replacement can be a revenue disaster. If a machine breaks and you have to wait for service or send the machine back to the manufacturer without a replacement, you will be canceling clients or scrambling to offer other treatment choices. This could have catastrophic consequences on revenue, client retention, and employee moral. If the manufacturer does not have a replacement machine offer to bridge the repair gap, you will most certainly need to have a contingency plan to avert the aforementioned consequences.

The equipment that a new start-up will be looking at typically includes treatment beds and chairs, the ancillary room necessities such as carts and lights, technology options such as LED, FotoFacial, microdermabrasion, and other facial equipment, as well as other more expensive items such as tubs.

Treatment Beds and Ancillary Equipment

The cost of the spa equipment will vary quite a bit, depending on the features; for example, a bed can be manual or electric. Know exactly what you are getting for the price. What does it include? Think of the details and be sure that you are comparing "apples to apples" when comparison shopping. Remember, the old adage "you get what you pay for" is really true. Also, remember that the client usually has to be in the bed for an hour, so it must be comfortable. Get in the bed and try it out. Does it feel steady? Comfortable?

Carts and lights are vitally important to the aesthetician. These small investments make the treatment processes more efficient and professional. Whether the light is attached to the cart or is freestanding is a matter of preference. The cart should have at least three shelves, and it is really helpful to have hanging side slots on the cart. Stools and chairs should be comfortable and steady. The wheels should roll without any impediment.

Remember that the beds, carts, stools, and chairs help make the treatments smooth and professional. Try the equipment on the trade show floor and make sure it works for you.

Technology Options

There are so many technology options available. Included in the "high tech" category are LED, FotoFacials, and hair removal technology. Other important forms of technology include galvanic, ultrasound, microdermabrasion, and steam units, as well as heat masks.

Each of these technologies will have many manufacturers and vendors. Use caution and investigate the companies and technology before making a commitment that could be financially disastrous to the company.

LED

LED, or light emitting diodes, is the newest technology craze hitting the spa. Used in the treatment of acne and aging skin, as well as for lines and wrinkles or cellulite, LED can be used as an independent treatment or combined with other treatments to improve the ultimate result. LED should be a standard treatment option in the spa.

Photofacials

Photofacials or FotoFacials are used to treat the color of the face, both red and brown. Red is associated with telangiectasia and brown with melasma or solar damage. It is an expensive machine that is a high ticket treatment for the client. However, FotoFacial is becoming a standard treatment in the spa and one that should be considered in order to compete with other spas.

Computer Programs

Computer programs are an absolute necessity to efficiently and profitably run the spa. Whether the spa has two aestheticians or is a multiple room spa with many aestheticians as well as other professionals, a computer program is an important aid in running the business. When investing in a computer program, look carefully at several choices. Make sure that it will provide all of the information that is needed for marketing, that the scheduling program will work for your environment, that inventory can be monitored, and that production indicators can be pulled without difficulty.

Every sales representative will tell you, "this is the very best price." But sales reps have the ability to make deals to drive business. Buying spa equipment is a little like buying a car. Be sure you get all the extras you can. But do not get duped into paying for something you do not want or need.

"Wear-and-tear," changes in technology, and flexibility are all considerations when evaluating finance options. Once you have all the information in place for the purchase, talk with your accountant to be sure you are making the best deal for your company. A professional opinion on subjects like these can keep you out of financial trouble.

■ HIRING AND TRAINING

Hiring staff is a necessary but time-consuming process that begins with reviewing resumes. Typically each business manager has a specific process for reviewing resumes, but a systematic approach will make it easier. It has been shown that only 1 in 20 resumes will convert to an interview. What is it that makes that one resume stand out? Why will you look at one resume over another? Those resumes that attract the eye are typically visually enticing. Their structure is clean, symmetrical, and simple, and they include white space that makes reading the information easy. The font use is consistent as is the use of italics, capital letters, or boldface. Finally, as a manager or business owner you are looking for a resume without any errors. This would include errors in spelling, typography, and grammar. Once the resume is scanned for information, the reader can hone in on the information that is important to him or her: experience, education, proximity to the spa, references, or other information.

Once a hire is made, it is time to train. Knowing who to train in what procedures can be straightforward in small facilities that have few available or qualified staff members. But in larger facilities, where there are several qualified clinicians, it will be a part of the business plan and part intuition to select how many or which staff members you should train. You might think that having every staff member trained in every procedure will allow more procedures to be performed. However, unless the volume of spa business allows all qualified clinicians to remain busy, you will have many people performing few procedures. As you now know, certain spa treatments are highly technique-sensitive, meaning the more you do, the better you get.[1] When adding a specialized or signature treatment, until client volume warrants training additional staff, limit the training to a few individuals who are your spa "experts." This limitation will also make your clients feel that they are getting this treatment from the most qualified staff.

While creating an expert will be cost effective during the delicate introductory period, it is not without potential disadvantages. Concentrating spa training to a limited few risks the possibility of client defection should that staff member leave. While noncompete clauses, penalties, and threat of legal action can discourage departing staff from pilfering the client list, the fact of the matter is that clients have a right to transfer care. They will be less likely to do so, however, if they receive various other services from other staff members, thus spreading around the loyalty.

Reading a Resume

As a business owner who will be reading a lot of resumes, you should look for several items on the resume that often will be indicative of a quality employee. Begin by noting the proximity of his or her residence to the spa's location. While it is always great to hire someone who has fantastic qualifications and experience, if he or she lives more than half an hour away from the spa, eventually the commute becomes overwhelming. The cost of gas, the time away from family, and the wear and tear on the car simply become too much. So begin with an understanding of where he or she lives. Once the resumes are evaluated according to location, next review the candidates' education, especially the aesthetic education. Did they attend a reputable aesthetic school? Do they mention how well they did in school? If not, ask. Also, look for any college education, even if they did not graduate.

As you continue to analyze the resumes, look for community involvement or hobbies. On first blush, this may not seem important. But what we know about a good aesthetician is that his or her life is balanced, that he or she has a family to go home to or a commitment in the community. These life commitments seem to keep individuals from creating unnecessary disruption in the office.

Finally, look for experience. Depending on your philosophy and training processes, this may be the least important factor in hiring someone. Rather you want someone who is grounded, smart, and presentable, and who has good communication skills.

Interviewing

Interviewing is an art form, one that many business owners are not very good at. It is important to realize that the more talking that you do, the less you will find out about the person you are interviewing. The objective of the interview is to find out as much as is legally possible about the person you are considering hiring. Ask questions that are legal and open ended. You will not find out much information with "yes" or "no" questions. Finally, get a "gut feel" for the person, and let your intuition have some power over your decision.

Making an Offer

Any offer made to an individual for a job should be in writing. It should have the information that is pertinent to the job, for example, the wages, the benefits, the hours, any probationary time, and the training. The offer letter should also include the start date and the location of the job.

Training Programs

Training programs should begin with basic information and progress to more advanced information. Training programs should not be tailored to the needs of a single individual; rather the training programs should reflect the needs of the facility. Typically, the training begins with a review of skin anatomy and physiology followed by the specific treatments that are done in the spa.

clinic protocols
written directives of procedure processes

The course should require familiarity with **clinic protocols** and the variety of available treatments and programs available in the spa. Once the student completes the classroom work and has passed the recommended examination, she can move on to hands-on spa training.

The spa training program should focus on technique. Critical to the aesthetician's success is the ability to replicate the treatments. The ability to reproduce a treatment comes with practice, and therefore extra time should be built into this arm of the training process. The aesthetician should not provide treatments to clients until he or she has completed a thorough training program. The definition of a thorough training program is often left to individual spas rather than the industry at large. This is because advanced programs still remain in their infancy. That said, any spa providing advanced treatments should carefully plan the presentation in the classroom, which should take between three and five days, and the practical experience. Practical experience can take up to one month before an aesthetician has provided enough model treatments and viewed enough procedures to be considered qualified to treat clients.

Example of Training Protocol—Microdermabrasion Protocol

Standard Policy and Procedure

Facial Aesthestics

Training and Certification for Microdermabrasion

Date of Origination: June 1996

Creator: Pamela Hill, R.N.

Date of Review: June 1997

Revisions by: S. Smith, M.E.

Date of Revisions: June '98, June '99, June '00, June '01, June '02, June '03

Policy #: 01-001

Attachments: Policy and Procedure Document for Microdermabrasion, Certificates of Completion, Written Test, Clinical Test

Title of Policy: Training and Certification for Microdermabrasion

Policy: All clinical staff will be licensed and insured in the state of employment. Certification through the company training program is required prior to patient care.

Purpose: To ensure that all clinical staff employed by the company are properly trained and certified in the techniques, policies, and procedures through the company training programs.

Scope: All clinical personnel

Definition: Clinical Aesthetic Personnel

Procedure Indications: All clinicians seeking certification will be recommended to the training program by their supervisors.

Procedure Contraindications: Not applicable

Required Paperwork: "Recommendation for Training # PER- 22" signed by the clinician supervisor

Testing if Necessary: Score of 80 percent or greater on the written examination is required before proceeding to clinical training. A score of 90 percent or greater on the clinical examination is required to treat patients.

Required Reading: Articles and technical information, provided by the instructor.

Classroom Training: The training will consist of two classroom days. The curriculum for these days includes a review of anatomy and physiology of the skin, wound healing, principles and techniques of microdermabrasion, and home-care regimens for microdermabrasions. A written test will be administered at the conclusion of the two-day classroom course. A score of at least 80 percent is required to move to the clinical training.

Clinical Training: The clinician will be responsible for finding 25 models on whom to practice the microdermabrasion treatment. These models should have different skin types and different skin problems. It is preferable that the models have not had any previous skin care or treatments. A full consultation is done followed by a treatment. The clinician will need to prove competency in consultation skills, the development of home programs, and the techniques of microdermabrasion described in the policy and procedure document. A passing score of 90 percent is required on the clinical training to be released to treat patients.

Clinician Requirements: Licensed professional

Clinician Required Training: Certificate of completion in a microdermabrasion course with a state recognized school or company training program.

Vendor Training

The training process for any technology should not be left to the machine vendor. The vendor is a good resource of information about how a particular machine functions and how to troubleshoot problems. The depth of necessary knowledge for treatments cannot be satisfactorily achieved with a vendor educator. However, the vendor typically has nurses or aesthetician educators that can speak from their experience and give information about treatments in the spa setting. It is this person whom you would want to speak with regarding complications, protocols, and near term or long term results.

■ UNDERSTANDING THE FINANCIAL STATEMENTS

income statement
the financial statement that summarizes the revenues generated and the expenses incurred by an entity during a period of time

balance sheet
document that states a business's assets and liabilities on a given date

Financial statements are the documents that should be produced each month reflecting your business's performance. These include the **income statement**, the **balance sheet**, and any indicators and goals that the business looks at on a regular basis.

The income statement is the document that presents the income the company has generated in a specific month and all of the expenses associated with that income. Understandably then, it will tell the story of where the money went and how much, if any, is left. This is an important document to revenue for the management of expenses, growing the income and increasing the revenues.

The balance sheet shows the value of the business. It reflects the long and short term debt and liabilities as well as the assets of the company. The balance sheet is a more difficult document for the average business owner to understand, but it is more important to the financial institutions you will be dealing with. Therefore, learning to read and understand the balance sheet will help you to become a more savvy business owner.

The indicators should be reviewed daily, weekly, and monthly. This information allows the business owner to hone in on a specific category of the business, for example, revenue per ticket, for analysis. Indicators are extraordinarily important to a well run business.

Whether you are an individual renting a booth or a director of a multisite business, you may feel that money always slips through your fingers. Reviewing the income statement monthly and the indicator hotsheet daily will help you to avoid some of this frustration. When you review these documents, be sure to evaluate them against your budget. Budgeting is the discipline you create to ensure that the money goes to the categories you want and does not ooze out into other places. But, sometimes it seems that despite your best efforts you cannot direct the flow of cash. This usually means that you have a flawed budget or that costs are out of control. If this is happening, you may need to have a professional accountant look at the books and help you to locate the problem. Keeping money where it belongs requires discipline and daily evaluation. Doing so will bring ultimate financial success.

Reading Income Statements

The income statement is an important document. It is one of the documents a bank will ask to see when you are getting a loan or lease. It is also a document that you should review monthly. Review the **indicator hot-sheet** in tandem with income statements.

Learning to read an income statement is easy. Start at the top, and look at the revenue or income line, which tells you how much money you have made. It includes all the package treatments redeemed, but should not include the revenue from packages sold—that revenue goes on to the balance sheet in a category called **deferred revenue**. The revenue line can and should be broken into different types of revenue: facials, peels, spa, etc., so that you know how much money you collected in each category. The next line is **cost of goods sold** (COGS); these are the direct costs and, like the revenue, should be broken into categories that respond to the revenue. The next line should be gross margin. Gross margin is the amount of money you made before **overhead costs**. General costs should include personnel, marketing, rent, telephone, and a general category. Finally, you come to a line called "income before taxes." This is the amount of money you really made before paying Uncle Sam. A good computer system will allow you to look at the aforementioned categories with a percentage attached. This is important because it helps you to understand the ratios at which the company is performing.

Cost Analysis and the Spa

Conducting a comprehensive cost analysis is important for the facility and the business owner alike. In order to make money, you have to understand how much it will cost to provide the procedure to your clients. Cost analysis has two separate components: **direct costs** and **indirect costs**. The first, direct cost, is a breakdown of all the costs that are directly related to implementing a spa procedure, in other words, all costs that are incurred exclusively by the spa treatment. These costs are offset only by payments of clients who receive this treatment. It can be confusing, so let us try to make it simple with some examples.

indicator hot-sheet
daily or weekly progress report that measures and provides daily insight into a business's or employee's performance

deferred revenue
money that the organization has received, but has not yet earned as of the closing date on the balance sheet; the amount is carried as a liability until the organization provides the goods or services for which the money was received

cost of goods sold
(COGS) directs costs of materials used in the products a business makes or sells

overhead costs
indirect costs

indirect costs
costs necessary for the functioning of the organization as a whole, but that cannot be directly assigned to one service or product

direct costs
costs that are directly and exclusively attributable to a specific product or service

The revenue on the income statement does not match the cash to the bank. Revenue on the income statement will reflect all treatments including redeemed package visits, which do not have cash attached because the package is generally prepaid.

indicators
key values used to measure performance over time as it relates to an organization's goal progress

Direct Costs

As we have stated, *direct costs* are those costs associated directly with the procedure. Let us use the example of microdermabrasion. In this case the direct costs include the cost of the regular purchase of crystals, disposable tips, filters, reservoirs; maintenance expenses; specific marketing for the spa procedure; and costs associated with training, insuring, and compensating applicable employees. In other words, directs costs are those that you incur solely due to the microdermabrasion treatment. Costs are always changing and usually increasing. You need to evaluate your costs at least every six months to make sure they did not go up.

Indirect Costs

Indirect costs are those costs that are not directly related to providing the treatment. Examples of the indirect costs are rent, telephone, or office supplies, and these should be considered in pricing. An indirect cost per hour of operation will help the business manager to understand how much it will cost just to open the door each day before any treatments begin.

Understanding the Balance Sheet

The balance sheet is the partner document to the income statement. Banks like this document because it tells them about your value: your assets and your liabilities. When you look at the balance sheet, the first category is usually the assets, which include equipment you own, cash in the bank, and other assets. The next page is the liabilities, which list the company debt. The balance sheet is a detailed snapshot of the company and helps anyone valuing the business clarity on its status.

■ INDICATORS AND GOALS

Company history speaks to not only the traditional history, such as "this is where we came from and this is what we look like now," but also the comparatives of **indicators** and goals. While these categories may initially feel financial in nature, the reality is that indicators and goals really speak to history and the ability to exceed the historical goals.

Setting goals for the facility and the aesthetician alike is appropriate. The goals should reflect the number of client calls, the number of clients scheduled, the number of clients treated, the referral patterns, and other important indicators for the facility. These goals should translate directly into the revenue goal for the facility.

Indicator Sheet

	Week One	Week Two	Week Three	Week Four	Actual	Goal
Number of new clients booked						
Number of clients seen						
Number of clients rebooked (after treatment)						
Number of packages sold						
Revenue per ticket						
Service revenue per ticket						
Product revenue per ticket						

The goals you set up should be attainable; otherwise everyone gets discouraged. Failure is a bad feeling, and one that you do not want in your facility, so be realistic. Also, if the goal is not being met, perhaps it was overshot and needs to be readjusted to achieve success. There is not anything wrong with adjusting goals just as long as it does not happen all the time. Setting goals can be an art. For example, if a procedure is being brought into an already established facility, the goals can be a little more aggressive because you have an already established client base. If, on the other hand, your facility is a start-up, then conservative numbers are in order. Goals should be set for six months and evaluated monthly. This way you can determine how successful the process is and whether you need to add additional advertising or marketing to stimulate the number of visits.

Indicators track the progress of business goals. Daily or, at the longest interval, weekly reviews of each hot-sheet will provide you with daily (or weekly) goal progress reports.

Without a weekly or daily hot-sheet you do not have the opportunity for improvement. A hot-sheet for a spa might include the number of clients scheduled, the number of clients seen, the number of clients rebooked, the average ticket revenue, and the breakdown between product and service revenue. You also might be interested in the referral pattern. The indicator hot-sheet should be the tool to evaluate, redirect, and grow the business. Over time it will be the comparative you use to measure your progress. Indicator sheets are simple in form. They need only the information you are looking for and should not be cumbersome.

Initially you may find that daily review of indicators is not necessary. In that event, a weekly sheet will do. But do not extend this beyond one week because it is too easy to forget about the growth process. At the end of the month you will get the numbers and, if they are disappointing, at that point you can do nothing to improve the numbers for the month.

■ BUSINESS RECORD KEEPING

Record keeping is a broad category and includes business record keeping as well as record keeping for client treatments. The records that should be kept for a business can be extensive, but with the computers and programs available today it is much easier than in the past. An organized business should include many different *sets* of information, and each of these categories of information should be easily accessible.

Included in the financial information should be revenue history, inventory, purchases, AP (**accounts payable**), and AR (**accounts receivable**). Aside from the financial information, the business should have easily accessible files on insurance records (health and liability), lease contracts, rent contracts, human resources records, marketing files, and client **database**. Insurance should be reviewed regularly and increased as necessary.

Pricing Strategies

Pricing strategies sometimes may seem like they are part of the marketing plan; however, pricing is quite different and should be evaluated independently of marketing. The theories and implementation of pricing strategies can be very sophisticated. For our purposes we will focus on four distinct pricing strategies: price and costs, price and competitors, price and customers, and price and business objectives. These pricing strategies will drive your business objectives, compared to promotional pricing, which is an occasional "price break" that may be used to move overstock **inventory**, for example.

Pricing and Costs

A spa has to ensure the revenue it generates will cover the costs and yield a profit. There are several different pricing tactics that cover costs and should be evaluated based on different business models. In the spa sector, one usually thinks first of **premium pricing**. This pricing strategy uses high prices to communicate the uniqueness of the product or service.

The next type of pricing strategy that might be used in the spa area is **penetration pricing**. In penetration pricing the price is set low to allow access into the market by gaining market share. The costs in this strategy are at a break-even point or a loss.

Next is **economy pricing**. Economy pricing keeps all costs low in order to provide the lowest cost to the customer. This is a very popular strategy, made famous by Wal-Mart.

Product bundling pricing is a tactic that is commonly used in the spa. This is the concept of *packages,* although product bundling is more sophisticated than packages. This type of pricing combines multiple services, for example, microdermabrasion and facials, bundled together. For product bundling you look at the costs and determine how much discount can be taken in exchange for collecting the fee in advance. Product bundling can also help the facility to be efficient in scheduling and increase facility utilization by knowing the number of clients who have packages and predicting the number of clients who should be scheduling. While there are many other different types of pricings, these four are the most familiar and most commonly used in our industry.

Evaluate your business objectives for the year before choosing a pricing strategy. Your objectives might include maximizing profits, attracting new clients, achieving a revenue goal, preventing further competition, or maintaining your market share. A business could use each of these pricing models at different times in the year to execute its plan.

product bundling pricing
pricing strategy in which one or more products or services are combined and offered at a discount

Pricing and Competitors

Entrepreneurship and competitiveness are often synonymous. In order for competition to translate into success, a spa business owner needs to negotiate a fine line between pursuing an active interest in the competition and appearing to be a nosy neighbor. By collecting small amounts of information, you can catch a glimpse of what the competition is doing with pricing, menu offerings, and compensation. The ability to collect and accurately translate this information into useful operational information for your own practice is a valuable skill for sizing up your own practice. The processes by which you choose to "get the goods" obviously need not be extreme or invasive. However, being watchful of advertising, word of mouth, or public presentations should give a fairly complete picture from which to draw your conclusions.

Pricing and Customers

In retail business it is said that the price of an item is the price the customer will pay,[2] meaning that the price of a product is consumer driven. It is no less true in the spa business. An important first step in setting your spa prices is to understand your customer. Because spas can be competitive, your customers may have one procedure with you and other procedures at different spas. This is one of the few areas where a customer survey is recommended; however, elaborate data collection is not necessary. Pricing surveys should be focused on price sensitivities about procedures and product, as well as value. In our environment, perceived value tracks closely with the price the client will pay.

Surveys can be tricky to put together. Preparing the questions in a manner that does not influence the answer can sometimes be difficult. Therefore, surveys that impact significant decisions, such as pricing, should be prepared by a professional. Otherwise the information you get will be exactly what you thought it would be, because you asked the question to get the predicted answer.

Pricing and Business Objectives

Pricing to facilitate your business's growth and profitability is a smart business tactic. But, when companies drastically cut prices in an effort to attract customers, the end result can be disastrous. To avoid using desperate, last option pricing decisions (and suffering the subsequent consequences on your bottom line), consider implementing a **standard pricing policy**. A standard pricing policy is a document that is controlled by the spa director or spa bookkeeping department and is a list of all the prices. The initial prices are calculated through a mathematical formula based on cost and a specific mark-up percentage. When prices are increased, there is a standard price increase formula that is used. This is far more effective than saying, "What is spa ABC charging? Oh, let us charge 50 cents less."

Standard pricing policies help the company meet its **yearly business objectives**. The yearly objectives are part of the **annual business plan**, which is a complex document that includes a budget, a marketing plan, and a growth plan (which includes isolated development plans for specific services). It gives focus and depth to the business growth.

When a spa adds a service, creating an isolated development plan for the growth is insurance for success. When you use a model such as the one depicted here, you will want to make the information detailed and appropriate to your individual situation.

standard pricing policy
business document that outlines the specific price range of a given product or service, preferred pricing strategy, and circumstances during which each might change

yearly business objectives
part of the annual business plan that identifies the goals a business would like to attain during a given fiscal year

annual business plan
growth plan that outlines business objectives, marketing plans, and budgets for the period of one fiscal year

Making a profit is the number one reason for being in business. Otherwise you are a nonprofit organization or are out of business. Figuring out how to hold down costs, meet goals, pay bills, keep employees happy, and provide outstanding customer service can sometimes feel overwhelming. There is one particular strategy that ranks on top to keep a business moving forward, and that is revenue strategies or *how you price*. Understanding pricing strategies, how the competition prices, and what the market will bear in your client demographic requires insight, skill, and intuition.

■ BUSINESS RISKS

In our litigious society, merely owning a business (let alone having a staff and equipment) makes a business susceptible to risk. Each year a business should evaluate the potential business risks, which could be damaging to the earning power of a company. Among the potentially harmful business risks are government regulations, technology changes, the borrowing power of the company, and possible litigation. Make sure alternative plans are in place, should a company face a problem.

Liability Issues for the Facility

More than just malpractice, the spa is at risk for a whole host of potential problems. Among the concerns that the business owner should bear in mind are the following: property damages (even if you are renting), workman's compensation claims and lawsuits, injury to employees when they are acting on your behalf outside the spa (for example, on the way to the bank), or sexual harassment suits. These types of potential losses should be discussed with the business insurance agent. The possible loss should not be minimized.

Insurance Coverage for the Spa

Find a good insurance agent and stick with him or her. Typically, your CPA can guide you toward a good agent. Sending insurance out to bid is often not a worthwhile endeavor; insurance agents like to build a clientele just like a good spa does. Therefore, if your agent is good, his prices will be fair and the service that he or she provides will become an important long term business relationship. Insurance reviews should be done yearly and adjustments made accordingly.

■ PROFESSIONAL CODE OF ETHICS

As far back as the time of Moses and the Ten Commandments there has been a guide for right versus wrong, but even the Ten Commandments require interpretation.[3] Of course, life was easier then, and less interpretation was necessary. The large cities of our world often put us at conflict with our ethics and values because in cities we are exposed to more: more situations, more people, and more opportunities. Each new situation may force us to evaluate our ethics and personal values. These situations require reflection and evaluation, recognizing that there is more than one right and ethical answer. Acting in an ethical manner is a matter of importance for those in the personal care fields. The results of doing otherwise will impact your ability to create lasting relationships, ultimately jeopardizing your career. What are ethics, and are ethics and success mutually exclusive? Do you need to be unethical to be successful, or is it true that the more ethical you are, the more successful you will be?

The first question to ask ourselves is, "Why have a Code of Ethics?"[4] There are two categories of ethical codes: personal ethics and **professional ethics**, and each of these categories has subcategories. While they may overlap, each individual document is important. Individually,

professional ethics
a code by which you conduct yourself, promoting high ethical standards and professionalism

the code of ethics is a very personal document that discusses how you will live your life and what your priorities will be in daily decision making.

A Professional Code of Ethics, on the other hand, should be very public and well known to all in our profession, as well as to our clients. Professional ethics are the guidelines set forth to ensure that each patient or client who comes through your doors is treated with dignity and respect while maintaining a superior clinical treatment. Professional ethics are decided on a larger platform than individual ethics. Professional ethics affect not only the business owner, but the employees and the clients of the business. If aestheticians are to be considered members of the trained service professionals (sometimes referred to as allied health professionals) as our counterparts in nursing, social work, nutrition, or others are, then the standard of a Professional Code of Ethics should be included in the workplace. "It should discuss appropriate and inappropriate behavior, it should promote high standards of client care, it should be used for self evaluation, it should establish a framework for professional behavior and responsibilities, it should identify us and create an image of occupational maturity."[5]

Each of you has a base of principles or ethics that you live by each day. You know the right thing to do, and when you consider the "wrong thing," it ties your stomach in knots. But those are seemingly the easy problems. What about the grayer issues that go on in the typical salon, day spa, or medical spa? (See Table 10–1.) Consider the following example. A client comes in on Wednesday for an eyebrow wax. You have never met her before. In the interview she says she uses Retin-A® regularly, but over the past week has discontinued the product. She is getting married on Saturday and would like you to wax and shape her brows. You agree to do so, in the process lifting skin from both brow areas. What seemed so simple is now complex. Did she really stop using her Retin-A®? Does she use other products that might cause a problem? Did she offer any examples of previous experiences with waxing? Did you ask about previous experiences? Did you provide the procedure with the correct techniques? What do you do now? Do you refund her money? Give her a gift certificate? Did she accept part of the risk when she asked for the treatment? She trusted that you would take good care of her, knowing she had a special event. Is this an ethical dilemma? What is the right thing to do? While we wish there were simple answers, there just are not, even in the most apparently easy situations.

Each day the clinician checks in for work, there is the potential for ethical conflict between herself and patients, between herself and col-

Table 10–1 Possible Ethical Dilemmas	
Ethical Dilemma	**Possible Considerations**
Keeping a patient secret	Consider the legal and safety issues
Knowledge of a dishonest employee	Consider your reputation in the company knowing this information, and the "right versus wrong"
Patients complain about the treatments of another clinician in your facility	Consider the "greater good" for the company, the patient, and your reputation
Patients complain about rudeness of the front desk and phone staff	Consider the "greater good" for the company, the patient, and your reputation
Incomplete training	Consider the possibilities of your aptitude and the usual training process vs. the right and wrong of the situation
Patient unhappy with a treatment	Consider talking with the patient, resource your manager

leagues, or between the clinician and herself. Ethical dilemmas will present themselves in the strangest ways and tug at your soul. It will be important for the aesthetician to be aware of her own personal ethics, those of her employer, and those of her profession to help guide her through the daily landmines of professional and personal ethical dilemmas.

Conclusion

It may sound elementary, but the financial management of a spa is critical to the long term success of the business. Many of us are in the spa and aesthetic business based on our passion, not our business acumen. Understanding the basics of business is critical to your personal financial success. If you are not comfortable on this side of the business, be sure to find someone you trust and put him or her in charge of running the business. Ultimately it will make the difference between financial success and failure.

▶ ⟩ ⟩ TOP 10 TIPS TO TAKE TO THE CLINIC

1. Look for manufacturers with a well established reputation.

2. Consider a short term lease or purchase agreement, so there is flexibility to trade the equipment or upgrade when newer models come onto the market.

3. The more frequently the procedure is performed, the more expert the aesthetician becomes.

4. Be sure you have proper insurance coverage.

5. Recognize the potential risks for a spa.

6. Use goals to achieve success.

7. Use indicators to measure success.

8. Keep organized business records.

9. Learn to read financial statements.

10. Learn to read resumes and interview potential employees.

CHAPTER QUESTIONS

1. What are indicators?

2. How do you identify the indicators for a spa?

3. How do you learn about the demographics for a spa?

4. What are the four pricing strategies?

5. Identify the direct costs for a spa.

6. Why is marketing an indirect cost of a spa?

7. What are the other indirect costs of a spa?

8. What are income statements?

9. How do you keep money from slipping through your fingers?

10. Discuss writing a business plan to implement a spa.

CHAPTER REFERENCES

1. Brown, L., MD. (2003, March). *The cosmetic facility: The role of spa in skin care.* Available at http://www.skinandaging.com

2. Canada Business Service Centre. (2004, February 15). *Setting the right price.* Available at http://www.cbsc.org

3. Dobrin, A. (2002). *Ethics for everyone, how to increase your moral intelligence.* New York: John Wiley & Sons, Inc.
4. MacDonald, C. (2004, March 9). *Why have a code of ethics?* Available at http://www.ethicsweb.ca
5. MacDonald, C. (2004, March 9). *Why have a code of ethics?* Available at http://www.ethicsweb.ca

BIBLIOGRAPHY

Bauer, M. (2005). *Healing power of acupressure and acupuncture.* New York: Avery.

Bek, L., & Pullar, P. (1994). *Healing with chakra energy: Restoring the natural harmony of the body.* Rochester, VT: Destiny Books.

Brown, L., MD. (2003, March). *The cosmetic facility: The role of spa in skin care.* Available at http://www.skinandaging.com

Canada Business Service Centre. (2004, February 15). *Setting the right price.* Available at http://www.cbsc.org

Kluck, M. (2001). *Hands on feet: The new system that makes reflexology a snap.* Philadelphia, PA: Running Press Book Publishers.

Wills, P. (1995). *The reflexology manual: An easy-to-use illustrated guide to the healing zones of the hands and feet.* Rochester, VT: Healing Arts Press.

Glossary

A

accounts payable all accounting responsibilities associated with recording and paying all vendor related business expenditures

accounts receivable all accounting responsibilities associated with recording and allocating all payments received by the business

acetylcholine component of the parasympathetic nervous system that plays a key role in the body's nerve impulses

acid mantle the acid mantle is composed of sebum and sweat, and is considered to be the protective barrier of our skin, protecting us from certain types of bacteria and microorganisms

acneic having acne condition

acupressure an ancient healing therapy, originating in Asia over 5,000 years ago, that utilizes the fingers to depress key locations on the skin's surface to prompt healing within the body

acupuncture treatment that involves penetrating the skin with thin, solid, metallic needles that are manipulated by the hands or by an electrical stimulation to prompt healing within the body

adaptive immunity antigen-specific immune response as a result of exposure to the specific antigen; for example, chicken pox

adduction the ability to move inward

adductor group of muscles three powerful muscles of the upper leg that regulate adduction of the lower extremities

adipose cells cells that contain stored fat in connective tissue

agranulocytes nongranular white blood cells

ala a wing-like structure, particularly the outer ear

albumin a grouping of certain proteins such as those found in blood or egg whites

alpha hydroxy acids mild organic acids used in cosmeceutical products. AHAs "unglue" cells in the epidermis, allowing keratinocytes to be shed at the stratum granulosum, providing skin with a healthier texture

amino acids organic compound that contains an amino group and a carboxylic group

anagen phase hair growth phase in which growth is actually occurring

anastomosis the connection point of different parts of a branching network

anemia condition characterized by a deficiency in iron, which is responsible for transporting oxygen in the blood

annual business plan growth plan that outlines business objectives, marketing plans, and budgets for the period of one fiscal year

antagonist a muscle or muscle group that counteracts the motions of the agonist counterpart

antibodies component of the immune system that neutralizes antigens, encouraging long term immunity to the antigen

antioxidant facials focus on the symptoms of the prematurely aged skin using antioxidant products including vitamin C, vitamin E, hyaluronic acid, or other nourishing ingredients

aorta primary artery that carries blood from the heart to the auxiliary arteries of the trunk and limbs

aortic semilunar valve trio of valves that prevent blood flow back into the heart

apocrine sweat glands larger of the sweat glands, which are housed in axillary (under the arm), pubic, and perianal areas

aponeurosis the tendon-like structure that actually connects the tendon to the bone

appendages any anatomical structures associated with a larger structure; the skin's appendages include hair, glands, and pores

aromatherapy the use of essential oils in lotions and inhalants in an effort to affect mood and promote health

arrector pili muscle an involuntary muscle arising out of the skin; causes goose bumps

arteries network of tubes that transport oxygenated blood to tissues, organs, and cells

arterioles smallest component of the arteries that connects with capillary beds

atria the two upper chambers of the heart receive blood for reoxygenation

atrioventricular valves trio of valves that prevent blood flow back into the ventricles of the heart

auriculotherapy also known as auricular therapy (ear acupuncture), this is a form of alternative medicine based on the idea that the ear is a micro-system, meaning that the entire body is represented on the auricle (or auricula, or pinna—the outer portion of the ear) in a similar fashion to reflexology (zone therapy) and iridology (iridodiagnosis), and that the entire body can be treated by stimulation of the surface of the ear exclusively

avascular lacking in blood vessels and, thus, having a poor blood supply

ayurveda an Indian word that is translated as the knowledge of how to live

B

back facials facial treatments that involve cleansing, toning, exfoliating, masking, and massaging the back; they are similar to a standard facial and involve the same steps

balance sheet document that states a business's assets and liabilities on a given date

balneology the study of spa therapy, hydrotherapy involving the use of baths from the sea water, freshwater, or thermal springs

balneotherapy along with spa therapy and hydrotherapy, balneotherapy involves the use of baths from the sea water, freshwater, or thermal springs, and may include drinking the water

basophils granulated white blood cell

bicep brachialis fleshy muscle of the upper arm that is responsible for flexing the elbow and rotating the arm

bicep brachii the muscle of the arm that bends the upper arm and turns the hand over

bicuspid valve heart valve located between the left atrium and ventricle that regulates backflow between the two chambers

blanket wraps the application of a blanket after a treatment to maintain heat or to cool the body

blood pressure the tension against the arterial walls, read in contraction and relaxation

bloodborne pathogens any pathogens that can be transmitted through blood or bodily fluids

Bloodborne Pathogens Act legally enforceable as of July 5, 1992, was initiated to reduce the transmission of hepatitis B and other bloodborne pathogens

body wrap a spa treatment that uses blankets, cellophane, or other products

C

capillaries tiny blood vessels that connect arterioles and venules, and where gases and other substances are exchanged

cardiac fibers flexible cells that make up cardiac muscles; found exclusively in the heart

cardiac muscles muscle tissue type, found exclusively in the heart, and a key agent in the ability of the heart to perform

cardiovascular system the entirety of the heart and blood vessel system

career plan a plan used to describe one's professional career goals and how to achieve those goals

catagen phase intermediate stage in the hair growth phase

cellophane body wrap a wrap that uses a plastic material to aid in the penetration of the product through the principal of occlusion

cellulite dimpling of the skin caused by the protrusion of subcutaneous fat

Centers for Disease Control and Prevention (CDC) a governmental agency that conducts research on disease and implements protocols and policies to ensure public safety

ceramides a class of lipids that does not contain glycerol

citric acid an AHA derived from citrus fruit (e.g., oranges and grapefruit)

clinic protocols written directives of procedure processes

clotting factors specific proteins that act together in clotting; defects in specific protein changes result in clotting conditions such as hemophilia

collagen a water soluble protein found in connective tissues. Particularly, type I collagen forms a network in the epidermis, and it is credited with providing skin with its tensile strength and firmness.

collateral circulation additional circulation, side by side

confidentiality prohibits you from disclosing information about the client's treatment or chart to others and requires that you take precautions with the information to ensure that only authorized access occurs

contraindications any service or activity that could cause harm to the client

cornified hardening or thickening of the skin

cost of goods sold (COGS) directs costs of materials used in the products a business makes or sells

cost to acquire the average cost per new customer of any one marketing strategy

cross-selling the process of selling related, peripheral items to a customer

cylindrical circular

D

database an electronic compilation of extensive categorical information relevant to business processes, such as marketing or inventory

database an electronic compilation of extensive categorical information relevant to business processes, such as marketing or inventory

deferred revenue money that the organization has received, but has not yet earned as of the closing date on the balance sheet; the amount is carried as a liability until the organization provides the goods or services for which the money was received

dehydrated skin the result of decreased moisture content in the skin

deltoid triangular muscle found in the shoulder that raises the arms to the side

deoxygenated formerly oxygen rich blood whose nutrient load has been distributed and is routed back to the heart, via the veins, for oxygenation

depression an area of skin that is lower than surrounding tissue

dermal-epidermal junction (DEJ) superficial side of the dermis, connected to the epidermis by subcutaneous tissue

dermis the second layer of skin, which is responsible for attaching the skin to the body

desiccation removal of all fluids

desmosomes small hair-like structures in the spiny layer (stratum spinosum) of the epidermis

desquamation shedding of cells, such as at the stratum corneum

diaphoretic producing or increasing perspiration

diastole part of the normal rhythm of the heart during which the heart chambers fill with blood

direct costs costs that are directly and exclusively attributable to a specific product or service

disinfection eliminates pathogenic microorganisms on inanimate objects (except for bacterial spores)

dry skin a condition resulting from a decrease in sebum production

E

ear reflexology an ancient Chinese technique that uses pressure-point techniques on the ears to restore the flow of energy throughout the entire body

eccrine sweat glands smaller of the sweat glands, which reside all over the body

economy pricing the low pricing of a product or service as a means to entice costumers to buy

edema swelling resulting from excessive fluid buildup in tissue

effleurage the massage movement using the palmar aspect of the hand or pads of the fingertips to produce a soothing effect

elastic wraps bandages that can be rolled around a client and have an elastic composition, allowing you to achieve a tight and secure wrap

elastin connective tissues

electrolytes ions required by cells to regulate the electric charge and flow of water molecules across the cell membrane

elevation ability to rise vertically

endomysium thin tissue sheath housing the muscle fibers

eosinophils type of granulated white blood cell

epicardium inner layer of the pericardium that has direct contact with the heart

epidermis outermost, avascular, protective layer of skin

epimysium outer layer of connective tissue sheathing a muscle

erector spinae long muscle that spans the length of the back and neck; key component to upright posturing

erythrocytes red blood cells

exfoliation treatments effective for exfoliating the outermost skin cells, revealing a fresh and glowing skin tone

extensor digitorum longus thin, long muscle of the lower leg; responsible for extending the four smallest toes, and pronates the foot

external obliques outermost layer of muscle tissue lining the abdomen

extrinsic aging changes that are brought on by the effects of the environment and our choices relating to them, specifically sun exposure

F

facials treatments that cleanse, tone, purify, and stimulate or calm the skin

fango the Italian word for "mud"; a gray-brown clay-like compound is mixed with thermal water that is rich in salt, bromine, iodine, and a number of other organic components, such as algae and protozoa

fangotherapy the use of fango mud

fibroblasts cells that produce connective tissue

fibularis muscle group group of muscles that spans the length of the fibula in the lower legs

filaggrin synthesizes lipids (fats) that are thought to serve as "intercellular cement"; important component of NMF

filtration hot springs geothermally heated mineral water that is fed by rain water that seeps into the earth through faults and fractures

flexation the ability of a muscle or muscle group to bend a limb at a central joint

flexor the major muscle or muscle group that causes flexation

foot reflexology an ancient Chinese technique that uses pressure-point massage on the feet to restore the flow of energy throughout the entire body

footbaths water used to soak the feet

formed elements red or white blood cells or platelets separated from the fluid part of the blood

free radicals atoms or groups of atoms that have an unpaired electron resulting in a highly unstable molecule

frenulum a small tissue that anchors a mucous membrane to surrounding tissue

frontalis muscle that makes up the forehead

fruit scrubs usually refer to a mixture of an exfoliating granule and an alpha hydroxy acid used as an exfoliation product and work by dissolving the cellular cement that holds dead skin cells together, revealing a smoother, more even skin tone and promoting an increased cellular turnover

G

gastrocnemius commonly called the "calf" muscle; responsible for extending the foot and flexing the knee

geothermally heated by the earth

gluteus group of muscles muscle group that makes up the uppermost thigh and lowermost trunk

glycolic acid alpha hydroxy acid derived from sugar cane; it has a small molecular size that allows for easier penetration into the skin

glycosaminoglycans (GAGs) polysaccharide chains, most prominent in the dermis, that bind with water, smoothing and softening the surface from below; most abundant GAG is hyaluronic acid

goals general statements of anticipated business outcomes resulting from well-stated objectives

granulocytes type of white blood cells containing granules

ground substance consists mainly of glycosaminoglycans (hyaluronic acid, chondroitin sulfate, and dermatan sulfate); involved in maintenance and repair of dermis

H

hamstrings group of tendons at the rear of the knee

hand reflexology an ancient Chinese technique that uses pressure-point massage on the hands to restore the flow of energy throughout the entire body

healing baths water treatments to address skin conditions, joint, muscle, or stress related disorders

heart disease any condition that impairs the normal function of the heart and/or blood vessels

hemoglobin respiratory protein found in red blood cells, which aids in transportation of oxygen from lungs to tissues

hemophilia disorder characterized by deficiencies of clotting factors reducing the blood's ability to clot

hepatitis an inflammatory condition of the liver, caused by a bacterial or viral infection

herb wraps body wrap treatment that includes the soaking of the wrap in an herbal tea blend prior to applying to the client

herpes simplex an infection caused by the herpes simplex virus, indicated by painful fluid-filled blisters on the skin and mucous membranes

histamine an amino acid histidine, found in the body

HIV/AIDS acquired human immunodeficiency syndrome (AIDS) is caused by the human immunodeficiency virus (HIV)

hydrating facials restore moisture to the skin and are beneficial for dehydrated skin types

hydrocollators heating units that heat the wrapping linens to an optimal temperature

hydrostatic pressure means of devising fluid pressure by means of measuring the pressure imposed by an external force

hydrotherapy the use of water in treatments

hyperextension extension of a bodily joint beyond the normal range of motion

hyperpigmentation overproduction and overdeposits of melanin

hypodermis layer of subcutaneous fat and connective tissue lying beneath the epidermis

hypopigmentation a lack of pigmentation in the skin

hypoxia deficiency in the blood's ability to transport oxygen

I

income statement the financial statement that summarizes the revenues generated and the expenses incurred by an entity during a period of time

indicator hot-sheet daily or weekly progress report that measures and provides daily insight into a business's or employee's performance

indicators key values used to measure performance over time as it relates to an organization's goal progress

indirect costs costs necessary for the functioning of the organization as a whole, but that cannot be directly assigned to one service or product

initial lymphatics interstitial fluid that first enters the lymph system and becomes lymph fluid

innate immunity the resistance to disease that a species possesses at birth

insertion muscle end point

integumentary system (integument) the skin and its appendages (nails, hair, and sweat and oil glands)

intercostal muscles short muscles that fill in the gaps between the ribs, aiding respiration

internal obliques inner layer of muscles that line the abdomen

intrinsic aging changes that would occur over time without the effects of any environmental factors

inventory an itemized list of merchandise or supplies on hand

involuntarily acting without thought, by way of unconscious mechanisms, or by instinct

K

keratin protein cell found in the skin, hair, and nails; insoluble in water, weak acids, or alkalis

keratinization a progressive maturation of the keratin cell in the movement through the stratum corneum

keratinocyte any cell in the skin, hair, or nails that produces keratin

Kneipp Body Wraps envelops a body part with wet and dry cloths that are either hot or cold; effects are achieved through temperature, length of application, and additives

L

lactic acid an AHA derived from milk

lamellar granules control lipids that produce NMF

Langelier Index (or the saturation index) is a chemical equation that is used to diagnose the water balance and includes testing the water for pH, temperature, calcium hardness, and total alkalinity

Langerhans' cells cells intimately involved in the immune response of the skin

lateral located on the side

latissimus dorsal large flat muscles that span the back

leukemia disease of the bone marrow characterized by excessive and unwanted white blood cell proliferation

leukocytes white blood cells

ligature a tying or other binding mechanism

lipids fat or fat-like substances, descriptive not chemical

lymph waste clearing fluid that contains white blood cells and lymphocytes to the blood for future waste removal

lymph nodes small glands that store the wastes collected by lymphocytes

lymphatic drainage technique of manually flushing clogged lymphatic vessels and glands

lymphatic vessels tubes through which lymph flows through its network

lymphocytes colorless cells found in blood and tissue that work toward cellular immunity

M

magnifying lamp an illuminated lamp combined with a magnification lens that magnifies the client's skin, assisting the aesthetician in the analysis portion of the facial treatment

malic acid an AHA derived from apples

mandible the lower portion of the jaw

marketplace any environment where two or more people buy or sell a product or service

masks high active ingredients in gel or cream form normally applied in the final step of a facial

mast cells large tissue cells present in the skin that produce histamine and other acute symptoms of allergic reactions

maxilla the upper portion of the jaw

melanin pigment that protects skin from ultraviolet damage

melanocytes type of cell (in the epidermis) that produces the pigment melanin

melanoma a malignant, darkly pigmented mole or tumor of the skin

Merkel cells usually close to nerve endings and may be involved in sensory perception

Mission Statement a clearly stated objective of a company to describe its goals

monocytes large white blood cells that roam the blood stream neutralizing pathogens

moor mud a natural peat preparation, rich in organic matter, proteins, vitamins, and trace minerals, is known for penetrating the skin, influencing enzymatic and hormone activity

muds along with clays begin with the erosion of rocks, usually carried away by flowing water and deposits along with decaying organic material and sediments at riversides or at the bottom of seas and lakes; used in spa treatments to refine the skin

muscle fibers cylindrical, multinucleated cells that can expand and contract on demand

muscular system complex network of tissue that supports, moves, and postures the body

myocardium muscular tissue around the heart

myofilaments tiny tubules that make up the muscle tissue

N

nare the nose

nasolabial pertaining to the nose and mouth

natural moisturizing factor (NMF) compound found only in the top layer of the skin, which gives cells their ability to bind with water

neuromuscular junction point where muscles interpret nerve impulses into voluntary muscle movement

neurons nervous system cells that process and transmit nerve impulses

neurotransmitter chemical substance that transports nerve impulses across a synapse

neutrophils phagocytic white blood cells

O

obliquely situated at a slant

obstructive lymphedema swelling of tissues with lymph stasis

occlusion accentuates the effects, good or bad, of topical agents

organelles a specific location within the cell

orifice a hole or opening

origin point where a given muscle begins

OSHA the Occupational Safety and Health Administration

overhead costs indirect costs

oxygenated rich in oxygen

P

palpebra the eyelid

papillae projections from dermis into epidermis that hold them together

parafango a mixture of fango mud and paraffin

patchouli an essential oil derived from the leaves of the patchouli scrub

peat therapy uses peat mud and peat suspension baths in balneotherapy and poultices

pectoralis major prominent muscles of the upper chest

penetration pricing pricing strategy in which the price is set low to allow for introduction into an existing market

pericardium fluid-filled encasement surrounding the heart and major blood vessels

perimysium connective tissue that makes up muscle fiber bundles

peripheral edema swelling resulting from fluid accumulation in the lower limbs

pH a measure of the potential of hydrogen that is used to describe the level of acidity or alkalinity

phagocytes waste clearing white blood cells

pheromones chemical substances, the release of which may affect the behavior or physiology of a recipient

pilosebaceous unit hair follicle and accompanying sebaceous glands and arrector pili muscles

plasma fluid portion of blood in which clotting elements and formed elements are suspended

platelets a clotting element

platysma muscle of the lower neck

plexuses a network of blood vessels

postinflammatory hyperpigmentation hyperpigmentation that occurs after injury to the skin

postmitotic cells cells that have completed mitotic division

powering the client database in-house marketing strategy that involves innovative and detailed use of information already contained in a business database in order to increase traffic

premium pricing pricing strategy in which the price is set high to compensate for a high quality product, usually with a high production cost as well

pricing strategies process by which a business determines the best way to price its product or service in order to entice customers while allowing for profit

primary hot springs springs that are powered by magma chambers, miles under the earth's surface

primary lymphoid organs thymus and bone marrow

product bundling pricing pricing strategy in which one or more products or services are combined and offered at a discount

professional ethics a code by which you conduct yourself, promoting high ethical standards and professionalism

prone position lying with the front or face downward

psoriasis a chronic skin disease characterized by inflammation and white scaly patches

pulmonary circulation path deoxygenated blood takes to become oxygenated; in through the right ventricle, into the lungs through the pulmonary artery, and into the left atrium via the pulmonary vein

pulmonary valve valve that separates the pulmonary path from the right ventricle

purchasing structured process a business undergoes in order to acquire materials needed for operation

Q

quadriceps large muscle at the top of the thigh responsible for extending the leg

R

rectus abdominis horizontally paired muscles running down the length of the abdomen

referral programs in-house marketing strategy that rewards an existing client for referring a new one

rete-pegs anatomic feature that holds the dermis and epidermis together

reticular dermis sublayer of the dermis that connects the dermis to the epidermis and is home to the skin's appendages (nails, hair, glands)

reticulin a water soluble protein in the connective tissue framework of reticular tissue

rhytids wrinkles of aging

S

salt glow a type of exfoliation process

sanitas per aquas (health through water) originates from the Latin word "spagere" (to scatter, sprinkle, moisten)

Scotch hose a hose similar to a fire hose used in water therapy

sea scrub stimulates the circulation, exfoliates the outermost skin cells, moisturizes the skin, and reveals a fresh and glowing skin tone

seaweed baths baths that use micronized algae powder added to the water

seaweed wraps wraps that include application of a seaweed mask followed by a thermal blanket to seal in heat

sebaceous glands small glands usually located next to the hair follicle in the dermis that release fatty liquids onto the hair follicle to soften hair and skin

secondary lymphoid organs lymph nodes, tonsils, lymph follicles of the mucous membranes, and the white pulp of the spleen

semilunar valves valves of the arteries, preventing backflow from arteries into the ventricles

sitz bath a form of hydrotherapy that assists with increasing the blood flow to the pelvis and abdominal regions

skeletal muscles type of voluntary muscles that surround, protect, and move the skeletal system

skin turgor the flexibility of the skin

slough cast-off skin, feathers, hair, or horn

smooth muscles type of nonstriated muscles that lines hollow cavity organs, such as the stomach and bladder, and functions to aid their operation

soleus long muscle situated under the "calf" muscles

standard pricing policy business document that outlines the specific price range of a given product or service, preferred pricing strategy, and circumstances during which each might change

stationary circle light form of circular massage using the fingertips

stem cells unspecialized cell that gives rise to a specific specialized cell

sterilization the destruction of all microbial life by heat, chemical, or gas

sternocleidomastoids pair of muscles that serve to flex and rotate the head

stethoscope device used to magnify the sound of a beating heart

stratum basale the lowest layer of the epidermis. The statum basale (basal layer) houses germinal cells and regenerating cells for all layers of the epidermis.

stratum lucidum sublayer of the epidermis characterized by the appearance of granules and the disappearance of the nucleus within the skin cells

stratum spinosum sublayer of the epidermis intertwined with desmosomes

striated lined or ribbed

subcutaneous beneath the skin

supination to rotate a joint a complete 180°; for example, rotating the wrist such that the hand faces forward then backward

supine position lying with the front or face upward

synapse the junction across which a nerve impulse passes from the terminal to the neuron or neuromuscular junction

systemic circulation blood and lymph circulation from the heart, through the arteries, to tissue and cells, and back to the heart by way of the veins

systole part of the normal rhythmic heartbeat during which the filled ventricles pump blood out the pulmonary artery and the aorta

T

technique sensitive a procedure that is performed differently from aesthetician to aesthetician based on his or her experience and knowledge

telogen phase stage of hair growth during which the hair is at rest

tendons fibrous and tough fiber that connects muscle tissue to a bone or joint

thalassemia condition characterized by defective hemoglobin cells, resulting in oxygen deficiency

thalassotherapy the therapeutic use of the beneficial effects of sea water

thoracic duct the main duct of the lymphatic system, ascending through the thoracic cavity in front of the spinal column

tibialis anterior long muscle that runs the length of the tibia and maneuvers the foot

toners, astringents, and fresheners have a hierarchy that ranges from sensitive to dry to oily. Typically an astringent is the strongest, a toner is somewhat milder, and a freshener is the gentlest. Astringents are stronger than fresheners and toners and are usually reserved for oily or acneic clients.

tortuous taking a twisting, nonlinear path

training an educational course designed to complete a clearly defined objective

training protocol a standard that is developed to ensure that a treatment is performed properly

transepidermal water loss (TEWL) the process by which our bodies constantly lose water via evaporation

trapezius two flat fleshy muscles that span either side of the upper back, allowing for movement of the head and shoulders

traverse abdominals innermost layer of abdominal muscles

treatment table the table specifically designed to aid in offering treatments such as facials, body wraps, or massages

tricep brachii large muscle that runs along the underside of the upper arm and extends the arm

tricuspid valve heart valve that prevents backflow between the right atrium and right ventricle

U

understanding your client component of the business landscape during which a business evaluates and acquaints itself with its target demographics

understanding your competition component of the business landscape during which a business evaluates its competition in terms of pricing, procedures, demographics, and promotions

urticaria pigmentosa allergic reactions such as hives with a large number of mast cells

V

varicose veins condition characterized by swollen veins, most commonly in the legs

veins carry unoxygenated blood to the lungs

ventricles the lower chambers of the heart, which force blood either to the lungs for oxygenation or out to the body

vichy shower an overhead shower with adjustable water pressure used in body treatments

voluntarily acting upon free will, without instinct or coercion

W

water testing evaluates the temperature, hardness (calcium content), pH (acidity/alkalinity), and amount of free chlorine that is available to neutralize contaminants in the water, as well as any other chemicals that may be added

waterborne infections can be acquired in the spa if precautions to prevent the spread of pathogens are not taken

watersheds drainage divide or the area that separates or divides two drainage basins

watsu original aquatic spa treatment

Wood's lamp a black light that reveals variation in skin color according to skin condition and is used during the skin analysis portion of a facial treatment

Y

yearly business objectives part of the annual business plan that identifies the goals a business would like to attain during a given fiscal year

Index

NOTES

NOTES

NOTES

NOTES

NOTES

NOTES

NOTES

NOTES

NOTES

NOTES

NOTES

NOTES